Wafa Dahmani
Aida Ben Slama
Mehdi Slim

Cirrhotic cardiomyopathy

Wafa Dahmani
Aida Ben Slama
Mehdi Slim

Cirrhotic cardiomyopathy

Prevalence and predictive factors

ScienciaScripts

Imprint

Any brand names and product names mentioned in this book are subject to trademark, brand or patent protection and are trademarks or registered trademarks of their respective holders. The use of brand names, product names, common names, trade names, product descriptions etc. even without a particular marking in this work is in no way to be construed to mean that such names may be regarded as unrestricted in respect of trademark and brand protection legislation and could thus be used by anyone.

Cover image: www.ingimage.com

This book is a translation from the original published under ISBN 978-620-6-72512-1.

Publisher:
Sciencia Scripts
is a trademark of
Dodo Books Indian Ocean Ltd. and OmniScriptum S.R.L publishing group

120 High Road, East Finchley, London, N2 9ED, United Kingdom
Str. Armeneasca 28/1, office 1, Chisinau MD-2012, Republic of Moldova, Europe
Printed at: see last page
ISBN: 978-620-3-37217-5

Contents

1 INTRODUCTION

Since the initial description of the hyperkinetic syndrome in cirrhosis, characterised by an increase in cardiac output, a decrease in mean arterial pressure and systemic vascular resistance, much progress has been made in understanding the pathophysiology of this phenomenon (1-3). Cardiomyopathy   " is an integral part of this spectrum of circulatory disturbances.

cirrhotic cardiac dysfunction (CMC) is currently recognised as a genuine cardiac dysfunction associated with cirrhosis (4).

Although it was given its own name in the late 1980s, it was not until 2005 that diagnostic criteria were established by a committee of hepatologists and cardiologists meeting at the World Congress of Gastroenterology (WCG) (2). This new entity was then defined as cardiac dysfunction, occurring in cirrhotic patients, characterised by :

> alteration of the contractile response to stress,

> and/or alteration of diastolic relaxation,

> associated with electro-physiological abnormalities,

> all occurring in the absence of any known cardiac pathology.

Recent advances in echocardiography, such as tissue Doppler and Strain Speckle Tracking (Strain 2D), have led to a better understanding of general cardiac pathophysiology(5) . With regard to the heart in cirrhotic patients, the value of these new echocardiographic modalities has been the subject of a number of studies in recent years, but to date remains unclear (6,7).

The exact prevalence of CMC remains unknown, given that it is a latent phenomenon, difficult to recognise clinically apart from a physiological or pharmacological stress stimulus (8). Nevertheless, it is estimated that approximately 30-50% of cirrhotic patients undergoing bénéйaer hëpatic transplantation show signs of cardiac dysfunction (9,10).

Recent studies have suggested that this entity is a predictive marker of mortality in cirrhotic patients, particularly in the event of digestive haemorrhage or in the operative sequelae of a transjugular intra-hepatic porto-systemic shunt (TIPS) or liver transplantation(11-15). It is also thought to be involved in the pathogenesis of hepatorenal syndrome (HRS)(16).

Given its clinical and prognostic implications, CMC is often overlooked and deserves to be investigated.

It was with this in mind that we decided to carry out this project, which aims to :

> Determining the prevalence of CMC in cirrhotic patients treated in thepato-gastro-enterology department of the Sahloul university hospital in Sousse.

> Look for possible predictive factors.

> To study the correlation between electro-echocardiographic parameters and the severity of cirrhosis.

> To assess the contribution of new ëchocardiographic techniques in the positive diagnosis of CMC.

2 PATIENTS AND METHODS

1. TYPE OF STUDY:

This is a cross-sectional, analytical study тепёе between September 2016 and May 2017 in cirrhotic patients followed at the hepato-gastro-entërology department of the Sahloul university hospital in Sousse.

2. POPULATION STUDIED

2.1. INCLUSION CRITERIA:

During the study period, we included all patients with cirrhosis who were hospitalised in the hepato-gastro-entërology department or attended the outpatient clinic.

The diagnosis of cirrhosis was made on the basis of the anatomopathological examination of the liver biopsy and/or a combination of clinical, biological, endoscopic and morphological findings, including signs of hepatocellular insufficiency and portal hypertension.

2.2. exclusion criteria:

Patients with :

\> antëcëdents of cardiovascular pathologies (arterial hypertension, coronary insufficiency, valvular pathology modërëe a sëre, rhythm disorder or heart failure).

\> recent digestive haemorrhage (in the two months prior to inclusion)

\> a body mass index > $30kg/m^2$

\> sëvëre tiiK'mie (iK'moglobin < 7g/dl)

\> chronic ethylism in excess of 30g/d

3. DATA COLLECTION :

The data was collected using a pre-established synoptic form *(Annexel)* comprising :

3.1. SOCIODEMOGRAPHIC AND ANAMNESTIC DATA:

\> age

\> sex

\> co-morbidities

\> medications, in particular beta-blockers and diuretics

\> lifestyle habits: smoking and alcohol consumption

3.2. CLINICAL DATA :

• heart rate (Fc)

• systolic blood pressure (SBP), diastolic blood pressure (DBP) and mean arterial pressure (MAP), calculated using the formula:

$$MAP (mmHg)= (2xPAD + PAS)/2$$

• the characteristics of cirrhosis, including its etiology and possible complications:

• oedemato-ascitic decompensation,

• digestive haemorrhage,

• hepatic encephalopathy,

• hepatocellular carcinoma,

• hepatorenal syndrome (HRS): diagnosed and classified as type 1 or type 2 according to the criteria of the International Ascites Club(17)

3.3. BIOLOGICAL DATA:

Biological tests less than 3 months old at inclusion included:

> a complete blood count (CBC)

> a prothrombin rate (PT) and an INR (International Normalized Ratio)

> a liver panel: including transaminases (ASAT and ALAT), Gamma Glutamyl Transferase (GGT), alkaline phosphatases (PAL) and total bilirubin (BT)

> a blood ionogram including a natremia and a kaliemia.

> creatinemia as well as creatinine clearance, which was calculated by the MDRD 6 formula adapted for cirrhotic patients (18). Patients were classifiedës according to the stage of renal failure with reference to National Kidney Foundation (NKF) guidelines (19).

> plasma protein electrophoresis

On the basis of these data, the severity of liver disease was assessed by:

> CHILD-PUGH score *(Appendix 2)*

We defined advanced cirrhosis with a CHILD PUGH score >9

> The MELD score (Model for End-stage Liver Disease): this score is calculated using a mathematical formula incorporating the values for bilirubinemia, creatinemia and INR *(Appendix 3)*.

We used a calculator available on the internet to easily obtain the value of each patient's MELD score.

3.4. ENDOSCOPIC DATA:

All patients had undergone an oeso-gastro-duodenal fibroscopy (OGDF) which noted :

> the presence of esophageal varices and their grade according to the classification proposed by the Japanese Research Society for Portal Hypertension and modified by the New Italian Endoscopic Club (NIEC)(20)

> the presence of gastric varices and their classification according to Sarin(21)

3.5. ELECTROCARDIOGRAPHIC DATA:

An electrocardiogram (ECG) was performed on all patients. The QT interval was calculated for each patient: this is the time that separates the start of the dëpolarisation of the ventricular myocardium (beginning of the QRS complex) from the end of its repolarisation (end of the T wave).

The length of the QT interval varies inversely with heart rate, so correct interpretation of the QT interval requires correction for heart rate. This can be done using various formulae *(Table I)*.

Table I: QT interval correction formulae

Formulas	Equation
Bazett	QTc = QT /VRR
Hodges	QTc= QT+105
Framingham	QTc= QT+0.154 (1-RR)
Fridericia	QTc = QT/3VRR
QTc cirrhosis	QTc= QT /3.02^RR

We used the formula "QTc cirrhosis". **The QTc was considered prolonged above 440**

ms.

3.6. ECHOCARDIOGRAPHIC DATA:

Each patient had bёгайбё of a conventional transthoracic echocardiographic (TTE) examination and an echocardiographic examination in tissue Doppler and two-dimensional Strain (2D Strain) mode, performed by a single operator.

Echocardiograms were performed according to the recommendations suggested by the American (ASE) and European (ESE) societies of echocardiography (22,23).

3.6.1. Echocardiography equipment :

This is a VIVID E9 type machine equipped with a continuous pulse and colour Doppler, with advanced 4D quantification tools.

3.6.2. Study of systolic function:

3.6.2.1. Conventional ultrasound data :

> the thickness of the posterior wall (PP)

> the thickness of the interventricular septum (IVS)

> **Left ventricular hypertrophy (LVH) was considered in the presence of PP and/or SIV >11mm.**

> tëlë-diastolic diameter (DTD)

> Tei-systolic diameter (TSD)

> telediastolic volume (TDV)

> Tele-systolic volume (TSV)

> cardiac output (DQ), calculated according to the formula: DQ= HR*(VTD-VTS)

> the shortening fraction (FR), calculated according to the formula :

FR=(DTD-DTS)/DTD; Its normal value is 26 to 40%.

> the left ventricular ejection fraction (LVEF), calculated using the Simpson method.

3.6.2.2. Strain Speckle Tracking or 2D Strain data:

Our study focused on the global longitudinal strain of cardiac fibres. The normal value for global longitudinal strain (GLS) is -21.9±2.1%.

3.6.3. Study of diastolic function:

3.6.3.1. Conventional ultrasound data :

> the speed of the peak of the mitral E wave (E)

> the speed of the peak of the mitral A wave (A)

> the E/A ratio

> E-wave deceleration time (TDE)

> Iso-volumetric relaxation time (TRIV)

> the diameter of the left atrium (DOG)

> the volume of the left atrium (VOG); we have calculated the

VOG index VOG*body surface area

> >

The left atrium is considered dilated if : Indexed VOG>34ml/m^2

3.6.3.2. Tissue Doppler data :

> septal early diastolic peak velocity (E'septal)

> early lateral diastolic peak velocity (E'latdrale)

We then calculated the ratio (E/E') or E'= (E'septal+ E'latdral)/2

4. DEFINITION OF VARIABLES

4.1. BASED ON THE WCG 2005 CONSENSUS:

> **Systolic dysfunction (SD)** is defined as :

o LVEF<55%.

> **Diastolic dysfunction (DD)** is defined as :

o an E/A ratio<1

o a TD >200ms

o a TRIV>80ms

The DD is classified into 3 grades:

> <u>DD grade I</u> (or relaxation disorder): if E/A <0.8 with TDE > 200 ms

> <u>DD grade II</u> (or pseudo-normal profile): 0.8<E/A<1.5 with 160<TDE<200 ms

> <u>DD grade III</u> (or restrictive profile): E/A >2 with TDE <160 ms

4.2. BASED ON NEW ECHOCARDIOGRAPHIC TECHNIQUES:

> **A DS** is defined by :

o S_{LG} <-18%

> **A DD** is retained, according to the 2016 ASE recommendations, if more than half of the available parameters reach the *cut-off* values, in patients with a preserved LVEF.

The four parameters recommended to identify a DD and their abnormal cutoff values are

> E'septal <7cm/s and E'Eiteral <10cm/s;

> average E/E ratio > 14

> VOG indexë > 34 ml/m^2

> maximum speed of tricuspid insufficiency > 2.8 m/s

Finally, the diagnosis of CMC was made when there was DS and/or DD, depending on the ultrasound parameters used, with or without support criteria.

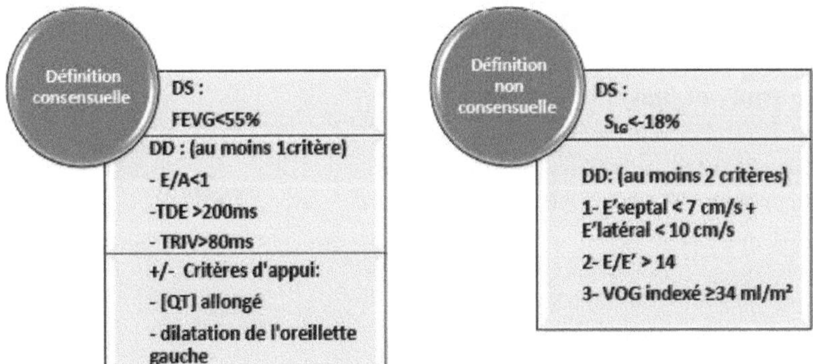

5. STATISTICAL ANALYSIS :

The data were entered and analysed using SPSS version 21 software.

For qualitative variables, we calculated absolute frequencies and relative frequencies (percentages).

The normality of the quantitative variables was tested using the Kolmogorov Smirnov test.

For quantitative variables that follow a normal distribution, we calculated means, ëstandard deviations and we dëterminë the extreme values. Elsewhere, we have calcиlë the mëdian and the interquartile range (IQR) 25%-75%.

The kappa index has ëtë been used to study concordance, which is interpreted as follows: between 0.81 and 1: excellent concordance; between 0.61 and 0.81: satisfactory concordance; between 0.41 and 0.60: moderate concordance; between 0.21 and 0.40: poor concordance; between 0.00 and 0.20: very poor concordance.

The link between 2 quantitative variables was ëtudiëe by the Spearman correlation coefficient (in view of the non-Gaussian distribution of certain variables).

The univariëe analysis procëdures were carried out where their applications ët were appropriateëes. Comparison of means was ëtë performed using Student's t-test for variables following a normal distribution, or using Mann Whitney U-test for variables with non-Gaussian distribution. Percentage comparisons were made using the Chi 2 and Fisher tests. All tests were ëtë rëalisës on independent ë samples of bilateral fagon.

In order to identify the risk factors linked<2s to event-independent fagon, we carried out a multivariate analysis using logistic regression, a step-by-step top-down method (in the first stage, we introduce all the factors whose "p" is <0.2 in the univariate analysis, and then, step by step, we remove the factor with the least significant "p".

A statistical significance level of 5% has been set for the various tests used.

6. ETHICAL CONSIDERATIONS :

This ëtude ëtait meiwe dans le respect du droit et de ^^ëд^Лë de la personne. It did not present any conflicts of intërëts.

All patients were informed of the scientific validity of the cardiac ultrasound and the absence of any consequences for their subsequent treatment.

Oral consent ëe^rë on the nature and purpose of the study was ëtë obtained from all patients.

3 RESULTS

1. DESCRIPTIVE STUDY:

1.1. GENERAL CHARACTERISTICS OF PATIENTS:

1.1.1. Number of employees:

During the study period, 109 cirrhotic était colllgës. However, 33 patients were ëlë excluded for the following reasons:

- ✓ Recent digestive haemorrhage: n=7
- ✓ Anemia sëvëre : n=6
- ✓ Arterial hypertension: n=12
- ✓ Coronary artery disease: n=3
- ✓ Rhythm disorders: n=3
- ✓ Moderate mitral insufficiency: n=1
- ✓ Chronic alcoholism: n=1

A total of 76 patients were included in the study.

1.1.2. Age :

The mean age of patients ëlaк 54±11.8 years with extremes ranging from 18 to 79 years. *(Figure 1)*

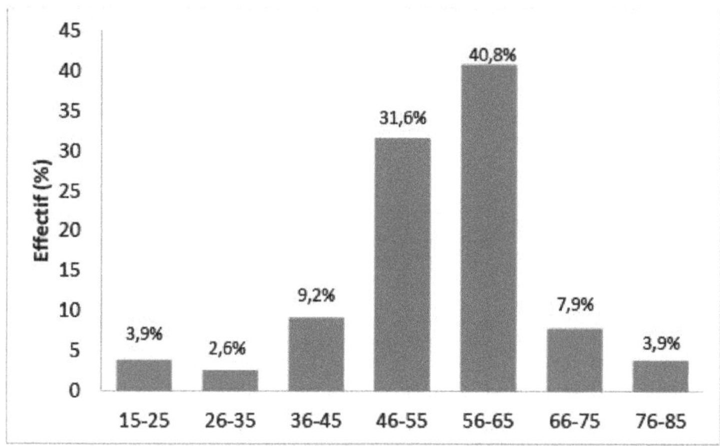

Figure 1: Distribution of cirrhotic patients by age group

1.1.3. Gender :

The study population comprised 45 men (59% of patients) and 31 women (41%) *(Figure 2).*

The sex ratio (male/female) is 1.4.

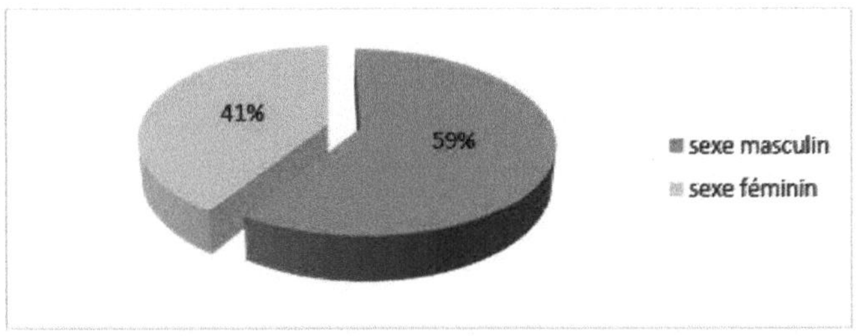

Figure 1: Distribution of cirrhotic patients by age group

1.1.4. Antecedents :

Twenty-two patients (29%) had one or more co-morbidities associated with cirrhosis. These were mainly type 2 diabetes, found in 7 patients (9.2%). *(Table II)*

Table II: Patients' medical and surgical history

Antecedents	Number of employees (n)
Medical	
Diabetes	7
Dyslipidemia	2
Ischemic cerebrovascular accident	2
Celiac disease	1
Autoimmune pancreatitis	1
Epilepsy	1
Surgical	
Cholecystectomy	5
Appendectomy	4
Gastroduodenal ulcer	2
Colonic neoplasia	1

1.1.5. Lifestyle habits:

Eleven patients (14.5%) were smokers, with an average consumption of 18 pack-years. Occasional alcohol consumption was found in 6 patients (7.8%).

1.2. CHARACTERISTICS OF CIRRHOSIS :

1.2.1. Circumstances of discovery:

Upper GI bleeding was the most frequent mode of onset (31.6%), followed by oedemato-ascitic decompensation (27.6%).

Table III shows the different circumstances in which cirrhosis is discovered.

Table III: Circumstances of discovery of cirrhosis

Circumstances of discovery	Number of	Percentage (%)
Upper gastrointestinal haemorrhage	24	31,6
Oedemato-ascitic decompensation	21	27,6
Cytolysis and/or cholestasis	14	18,4
Ictere	7	9,2
Abdominal ultrasound	7	9,2

| Thrombocytopenia | 3 | 3,9 |
| **Total** | **76** | **100** |

1.2.2. Etiologies of cirrhosis:

Cirrhosis was of viral origin in 35 cases (46%): post-viral B cirrhosis in 30 patients (39.5%) and post-viral C cirrhosis in 5 patients (6.6%) (Figure 3).

Elsewhere, it was alcoholic cirrhosis, cirrhosis of dysimmune origin, non-alcoholic stëato-hëpatitis (NASH) or cryptogënic cirrhosis *(Figure4)*.

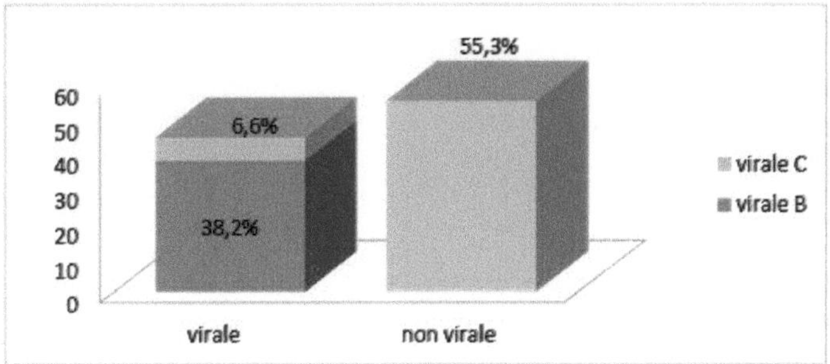

Figure 3: Distribution of patients according to viral or non-viral origin of cirrhosis

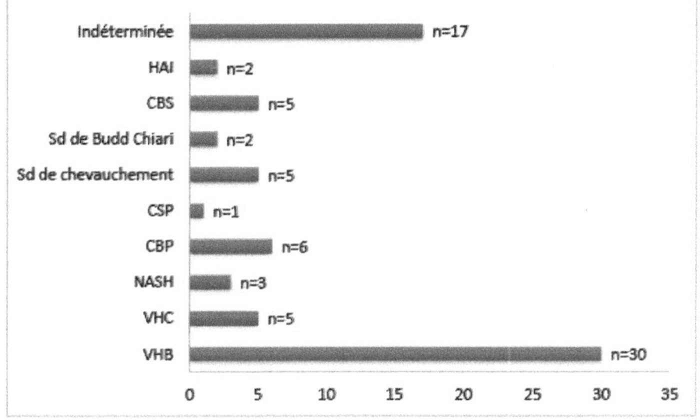

Figure 4: Distribution of patients according to cirrhosis etiology

(HAI: autoimmune hepatitis, CBS: secondary biliary cirrhosis, PSC: primary sclerosing cholangitis, PBC: primary biliary cholangitis, NASH: non-alcoholic steatohepatitis, HCV: post-viral cirrhosis C, HBV: post-viral cirrhosis B)

1.2.3. Biological data:

Anemia was found in 52 patients (68.4%), of whom 25(33%) had a hemoglobin of less than 10g/dl.

TP was greater than 50% in 30 patients (65%).

Twenty-two patients (29%) had cytolysis and 26 (34.2) had cholestasis.

Mean blood creatinine clearance was 94 ± 36.2 ml/min/1.73m^2 [16.1 - 191 ml/min/1.73m^2]. Eighteen patients (23.7%) had moderate to sevëre renal insufficiency. Renal function abnormalities are represented in *Figure 5*.

Table IV reports the various biological parameters of the population studied.

Table IV: Biological parameters of patients

	Mean value±standard deviation (or median)	Values extremes
Hemoglobin (g/dl)	11,1±2,1	[7,2-15,9]
Inserts (elements/mm)^3	100146±64036	[24000-310000]
TP (%)	68,2±16,4	[22-94]
INR	1,4	[1,04-4,95]
ASAT (UI/l))	59	[10-616]
ALT (IU/l)	42,8	[8-793]
Total bilirubinemia (umol/l)	48,5	[4-412]
GGT (IU/l)	96,4	[10-515]
PAL (IU/l)	164,7	[32-964]
Uree (mmol/l)	7,5	[2,1-30,1]
Creatinine levels (umol/l)	76,4±37,7	[35-316]
Creatinine clearance (ml/min/1.73m2)	94±36	[16-191]
Natremia (mmol/l)	136,3±3,7	[129-143]
Albuminemia (g/l)	31	[18-45]

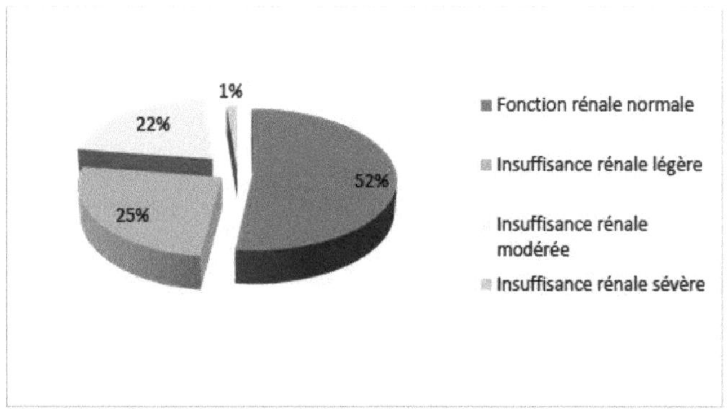

Figure 5: Distribution of patients according to renal function

1.2.4. Severity of cirrhosis:

> CHILD PUGH score:

Cirrhosis was classifiedëe CHILD PUGH B in the majority of cases (44.7%). Only 9 patients (11.8%) had CHILD PUGH C cirrhosis *(Figure 6)*.

A CHILD PUGH score >9 was found in 23 patients (30.3%) *(Figure 7)*.

CHILD PUGH score

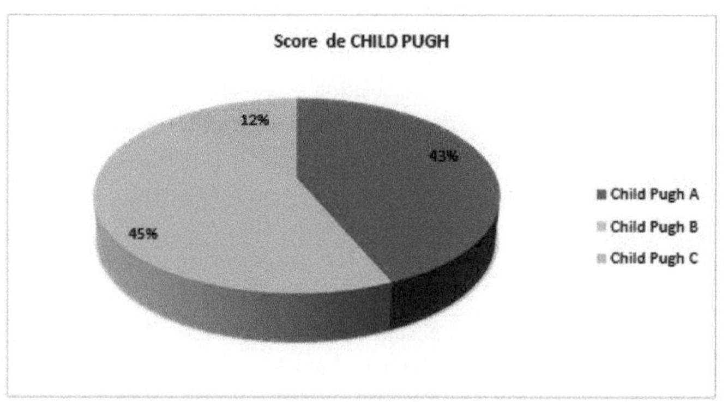

Figure 6: Distribution of cirrhotics according to the stages of the CHILD PUGH score

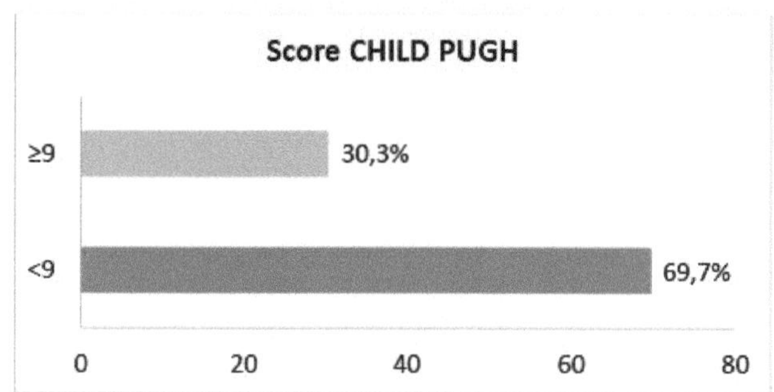

Figure 7: Distribution of cirrhotics according to Child Pugh score

> MELD score :

The MELD mëdian score was 11 with an IIQ27-75 [10 ;14].

The majority of patients (77.6%) had a MELD score of <15 *(Figure 8)*.

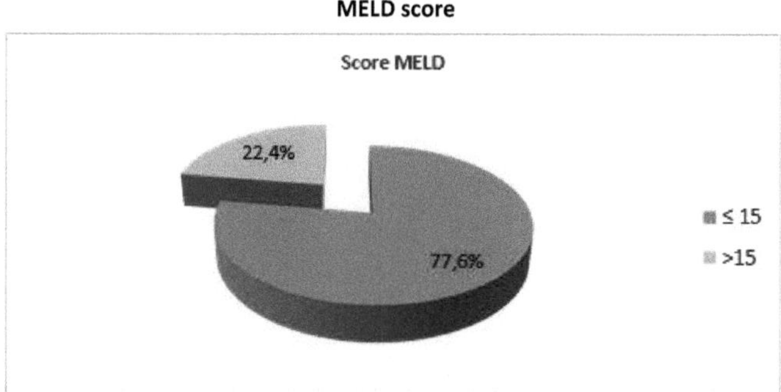

Figure 8: Distribution of cirrhotics according to MELD score

1.2.5. Endoscopic data :

Seventy-two patients (94.7%) had resophageal varices which ëwere classified grade II in 67% and grade III in 10%. The LVs had ë1.ë objectivees in only 12 patients (15.8%).

(Table V)

Beta-blocker therapy was prescribed in 64 patients (84.2%), as primary prophylaxis (60 cases) or secondary prophylaxis in association with elastic ligation (4 cases). The molecule used was Propranolol, with an average dose of 49 mg per day and extremes ranging from 40 mg to 120 mg per day.

Table V: Objective endoscopic signs of portal hypertension at upper gastrointestinal endoscopy :

Endoscopic signs of portal hypertension		Number of employees (n)	Percentage (%)
Esophageal varices	absent	4	5,3
	Grade I	17	22,4
	Grade II	48	63,2
	Grade III	7	9,2
Gastric varices	absent	64	84,2
	GOV1	5	6,6
	GOV 2	4	5,3
	IGV1	3	3,9

1.2.6. Abdominal ultrasound data:

Abdominal ultrasound showed collateral venous circulation and portal trunk dilatation in 55 (72.3%) and 36 (47.3%) cases respectively.

A splënomëgalie ë'!^^!. found in 57 patients (75%) with a mean spenic fkche of 15 cm.

1.2.7. Evolving complications:

Thirty-six patients (47.4%) had experienced one or more episodes of gastrointestinal bleeding.

Forty-seven patients (61.8%) had an antëcëdent of oedëmato-ascitic dëcompensation, 6 of whom were at the refractory ascites stage. At the time of inclusion, 25 patients (32.9%) had ascites, of whom 23 (30.3%) were receiving diuretic treatment (spironolactone and/or furosëmide).

A type 2 SHR ë1як found in 4 cases (5.3%).

Cirrhosis was dëgënërëe in 10 patients (13%). *(Figure 9)*

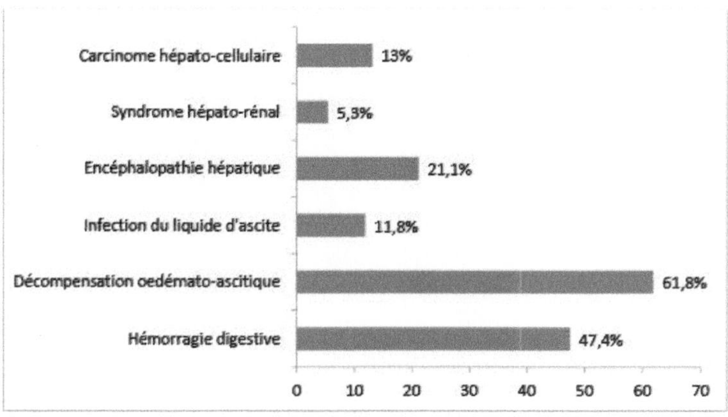

Figure 9: Distribution of patients according to the progressive complications of their disease

1.3. STUDY OF CARDIOVASCULAR FUNCTION:

1.3.1. Cardiovascular examination data:

The mean Fc was 67±11.9 bpm. It was 65 bpm for bëtabloquës patients and 77 bpm for non-bëtabloquës patients.

The mean values of the patients' heart rate, systolic and diastolic blood pressures and their extreme values are shown in *Table VI.*

Table VI: Hemodynamic parameters of patients

	Average value	Extreme values
Fc (bpm)	67±11,9	[44-93bpm]
PAS (mmHg)	110[100 ; 120]	[90-140mmHg].
DBP (mmHg)	70[60 ; 80]	[40-90mmHg].
MAP (mmHg)	81[73 ; 90]	[63-106mmHg].

Fc: heart rate; SAP: systolic blood pressure; DBP: diastolic blood pressure; MAP: mean arterial pressure

1.3.2. Electrocardiographic data:

The mean QTc interval was 434.5 ms, with extremes ranging from 380 to 494 ms. The QTc 6was aПопдë in 33 patients (43.5%). *(Figure 10)*

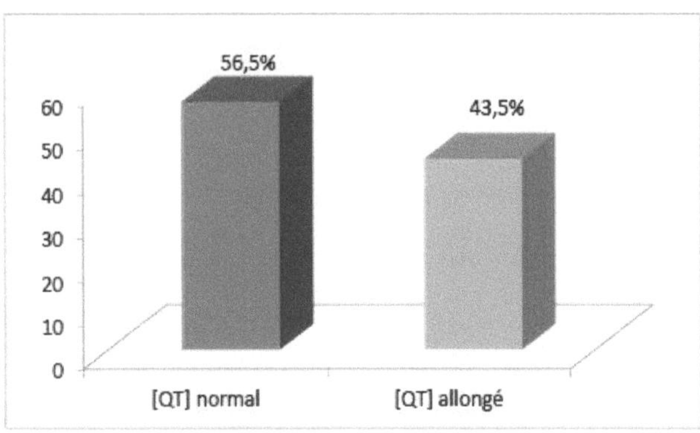

Figure 10: Distribution of patients according to QT interval

1.3.3. Conventional echocardiographic data:

1.3.3.1.   Study of systolic function:

LVEF had a mëdian value of 67% with extremes ranging from 50 to 75%. *(Figure 11)*

A DS (LVEF <55%) ëtait notëe in 4 patients (5.2%). *(Figure 12)*

FR and DQ ët were within normal limits in all patients.

In addition, LVH ëtait notëe in 12 patients (15.8%). *(Figure 13)*

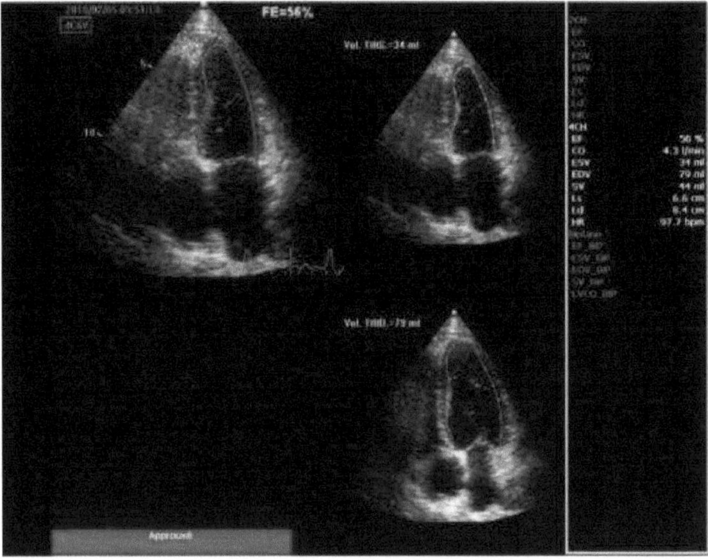

Figure 11: Example of automatic measurement of left ventricular ejection fraction

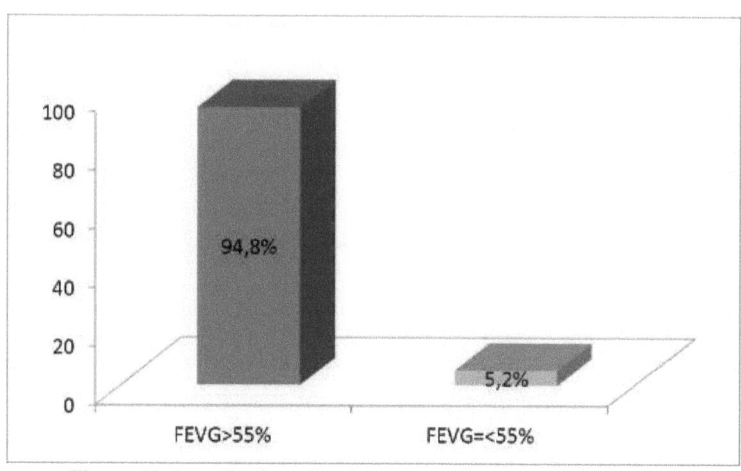

Figure 12: Distribution of patients according to systolic function

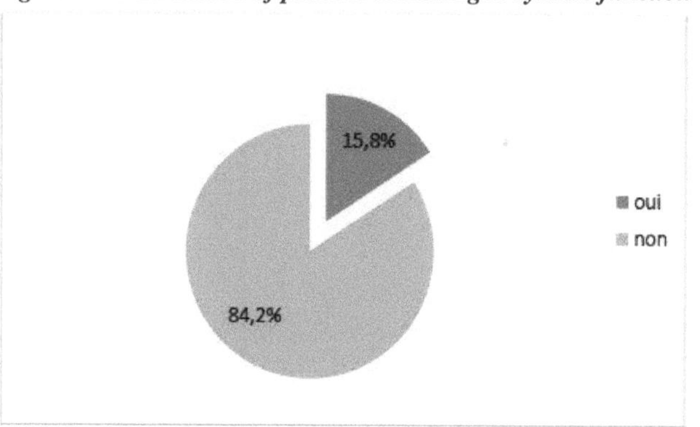

Figure 13: Distribution of cirrhotics according to left ventricular hypertrophy

1.3.3.2.   *Study of diastolic function :*

Diastolic function was studied on the basis of the mitral profile. *Table VII* reports the conventional ëchocardiographic parameters relating to diastolic function.

Table VII: Conventional echocardiographic parameters relating to diastolic function

Echocardiographic parameters	Mean values ± standard deviation
E/A 1.2 ± 0.5	
TDE (ms) 200 ± 64.6	
TRIV (ms) 91,5±23,9	

> An E/A ratio of less than 1 was observed in 32 patients (42.1%).

> A TDE >200 ms was noted in 30 cases, i.e. 39.4% of the population.

> A TRIV>80 ms was found in 33 patients (43.4%) *(Figure 14)*.

In all, DD was found in 39 cirrhotics (51.3%). The majority of these patients (74.4%) had a grade I DD indicating a relaxation disorder. *(Figure 15)*

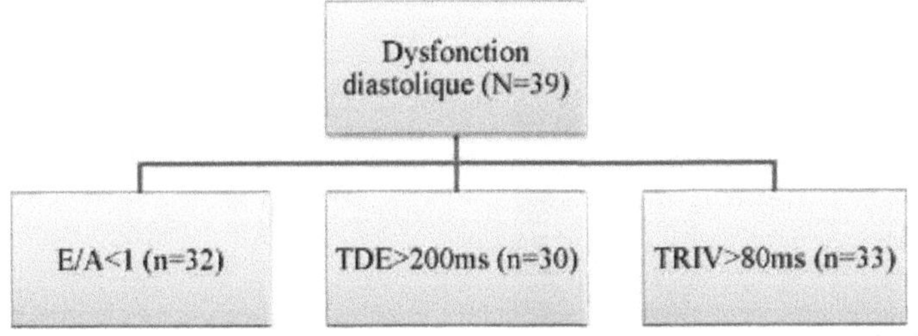

Figure 14: Prevalence of echocardiographic parameters defining diastolic dysfunction

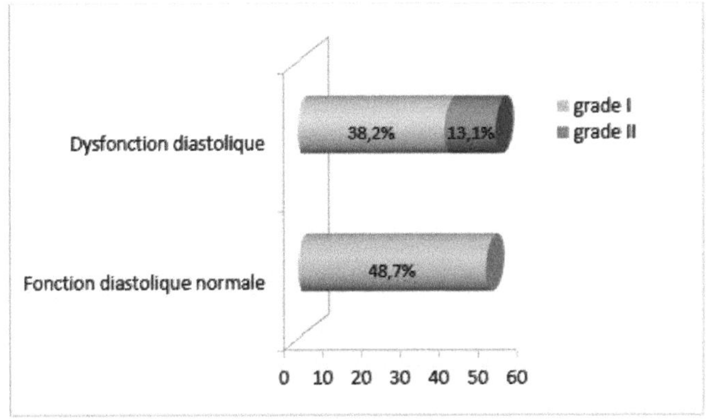

Diastolic dysfunction
Normal diastolic function

Figure 15: Distribution of patients according to diastolic function

1.3.4. Data from new echocardiographic techniques (tissue Doppler and Strain2D):

The main data from the new ëchocardiographic modalities are summarised *in Table VIII.*

1.3.4.1.   Study of systolic function:

A SLG<-18, tëmoignant of a DS, ëlaH rейоиyë in 10 patients (13.2%). *(Figure 16)*

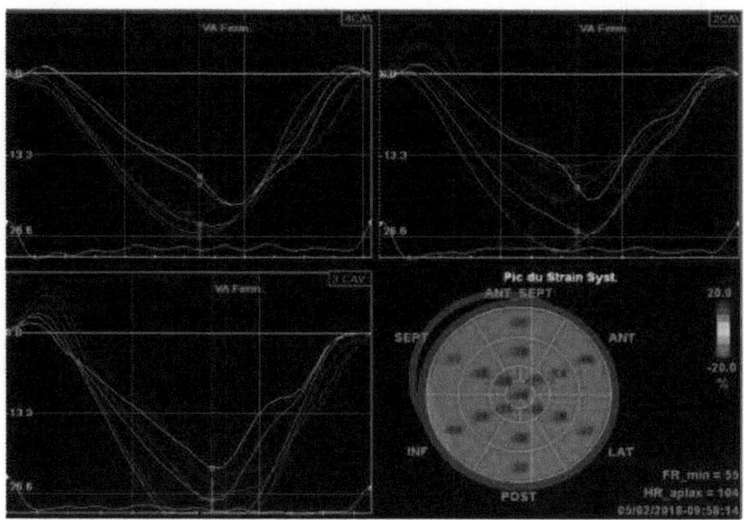

Figure 16: Example of a global longitudinal strain measurement presented in the form of a ba'uf diagram, accompanied by temporal strain curves and cutting planes.

1.3.4.2. Study of diastolic function :

The study of diastolic function by tissue Doppler showed a vëlocitë of the septal E' wave<7cm/s associated with a vëlocitë of the lateral E' wave- 10cm/s in 30 patients (39.4%).

An E/E'>14 ёляк ratio was found in 4 patients (5.3%).

In addition :

OG ёляк dilatation obserxes in 45 cases (59.2%), with a mean VOG indexë of 40.3± 6.6ml/m .^{2}

In total, according to the ASE 2016 recommendations, a DD ёляк found in 25 patients (32.9%).

Table VIII: Echocardiographic parameters of 2D Strain and Tissue Doppler

Parameters	Mean values ± standard deviation
Overall longitudinal grain (%)	-20,7 ± 2,3
Septal E' (cm/s)	8,2 ± 2,7
E' laterale (cm/s)	11,4± 4,2
E/E'	8 ± 2,5

1.3.5. Prevalence of cirrhotic cardiomyopathy in our population:

> According to the diagnostic criteria of the WCG 2005, we have notë

* Isolated DS in 2 patients (2.6%)
* Isolated DD in 37 cirrhotics (48.7%)
* DS associated with DD in 2 cases (2.6%)

A total of 41 patients (53.9%) were diagnosed with CMC. *(Figure 17).*

Among these 41 patients, QT interval prolongation and left atrial dilatation were noted in 21 and 15 cases respectively.

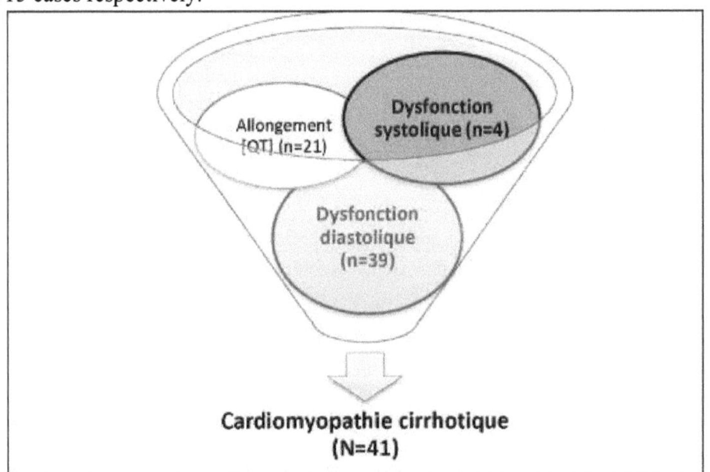

Figure 17: Electro-echocardiographic abnormalities in patients with cirrhotic cardiomyopathy (2005 consensus)

> According to the ASE 2016 recommendations and based on tissue Doppler and 2D Strain data, we found:

- Isolated DS in 6 patients (7.9%)
- Isolated DD in 21 patients (27.6%)
- DS associated with DD in 4 cases (5.3%)

Consequently, 31 patients had CMC, representing a prevalence of 40.8%.

Among these 31 patients, prolongation of the QT interval and dilatation of the left atrium were noted in 14 and 22 cases respectively.

2. ANALYTICAL STUDY :

2.1. CONCORDANCE BETWEEN CONSENSUS AND NON-CONSENSUS DEFINITIONS :

The kappa concordance index between the two definitions was 0.585, indicating moderate concordance (p<0.001).

Three patients who were considered not to have CMC had signs of DS and/or DD according to the new recommendations. In addition, 13 patients labelled as CMC carriers (according to the consensus definition) had normal LMS values and normal tissue Doppler diastolic function. *(Table IX)*

Table IX: Agreement between the two definitions (consensus and non-consensus)

		CMC (definition non consensus)		Total (N)	p
		No (n)	Yes (n)		
CMC (definition consensus)	**No (n)**	32	3	35	**<0,001**
	Yes (n)	13	28	41	

Total (N)	45	31	76

Furthermore, patients with CMC (according to the consensus definition) had lower E'septal and lateral vëlocitës and a higher E/E' ratio compared with patients without CMC; the differences ëtended to be statistically significant (p<0.001, p<0.001 and p=0.01 respectively). However, there was no significant difference in the value of SLG (p=0.11)*(Table X)*.

Table X: Comparison of tissue Doppler and 2D Strain echocardiographic parameters between patients with and without cirrhotic cardiomyopathy

Variables	Cirrhotic cardiomyopathy		P
	No	Yes	
LMS (%)	-21,2±2,3	-20,5±2,3	0,11
E'septale(cm/s)	9,9±2,3	6,7±2	**<0,001**
E'laterale (cm/s)	14,1±4	9±2,5	**<0,001**
E/E'	7,3±1,8	8,6±2,7	**0,01**

2.2. FACTORS associatedA THE CARDIOMYOPATHY CIRRHOTIC (CONSENSUS DEFINITION):

CMC was more frequent in women than in men (p=0.04). (Table XI)

Patients with a CMC ëwere older than those with no CMC with a statistically significant difference (51 years vs 58 years; p=0.01).

Biological parameters (transaminases, GGT, PAL, BT, TP, albuminemia, creatinine clearance) were comparable between the two groups of patients.

Furthermore, a CHILD PUGH score >9 was significantly more common in patients with CMC (p=0.002).

The majority of patients with a MELD score >15 (64.7%) had a CMC, but without reaching the significance threshold (p=0.312).

Table XI: Comparison of demographic and clinical-biological parameters between patients with and without cirrhotic cardiomyopathy

Variables	Cardiomyopathy		Odds ratio (IC95%)	P
	No(n=35)	Yes(n=41)		
Age (years)	51±11,7	58±11	1,042(1,001-1,084)	0,01
Gender Female n(%)	10(32,2)	21(67,7)	**2,62(1,01-6,824)**	**0,04**
Male n(%)	25(55,6)	20(44,4)		
Etiology of Non viral cirrhosis	20 (48,8%)	21 (51,2%)	1,27(0,513-3,146)	0,6
viral	15 (42,9%)	20 (57,1%)		
TakingNo	5 (41,7%)	7 (58,3%)	0,81(0,232-2,821)	0,74
beta-blocker yes	30 (46,9%)	34 (53,1%)		
MAP (mmHg)	8,4±0,9	7,9±1,1	1,059(0,952-1,064)	0,36
Fc (bpm)	65,4±10	68,6±13,4	1,024(0,984-1,065)	0,24
AscitesNon	23 (45,1%)	28 (54,9%)	0,890(0,341-2,322)	0,81
Yes	12 (48%)	13 (52%)		
Hemoglobin (g/l)	11±1,9	11,2±2,4	1,037(0,840-1,280)	0,7
TP (%)	67,8±18,1	62,5±14	1,002(0,975-1,031)	0,823

Parameter				Odds ratio (95% CI)	p
ASAT (UI/l)		44[26 ;41]	50[26 ;64]	1,004(0,995-1,014)	0,762
ALT (UI/l)		32[20 ;40]	26[21;40]	1,003(0,994-1,013)	0,857
BT (umol/l)		27[12;41]	26[14 ;52]	1,008(0,994-1,020)	0,595
Creatinine	**clearance<60 n(%)**	32 (55,2%)	26 (44,8%)	**6,154(1,6-23,579)**	**0,04**
(ml/min/1 .7³m2)	**>60 (n%)**	3 (16,7%)	15 (83,3%)		
Albumin (g/l)		34[27;37]	28,8[26;36]	0,940(0,869-1,017)	0,163
CHILD	**PUGH<9 n(%)**	29(54,7)	24(45,3)	**3,424(1,167-10,046)**	**0,02**
>9 n(%)		6(26,1)	17(73,9)		
MELD>15 n(%)		29(49,2)	30(50,8)	1,772(0,579-5,421)	0,312
>15 n(%)		6(35,3)	11(64,7)		

> We subsequently тепё a top-down stepwise logistic regression analysis to identify other indëpendent predictors.

> In rësumë we retained age, fëminine sex, and a CHILD PUGH score>9 as indëpendent predictive factors for CMC. *(Table XII)*

Table XII: Independent predictive factors of cirrhotic cardiomyopathy in logistic regression

Parameters	P	Adjusted odds ratio (95% CI)
Age	**0,039**	**1,050(1,003-1,103)**
Female sex	**0,044**	**3,006(1,029-8,778)**
CHILD PUGH>9	**0,015**	**4,363(1,328-14,331)**

3.3 CORRELATION BETWEEN SEVERITY OF CIRRHOSIS AND ELECTRO-ECHOCARDIOGRAPHIC PARAMETERS:

> Of all the ëchocardiographic ëtudiës parameters (reported^s by *Table XIII),* only the VOG ë1ш1: positively correlated with both the CHILD PUGH score (r=0.351 ; p=0.002) *(Figure 18),* and the MELD
(r=0.329 ;p=0.004*) (Figure 19)*

Table XIII: Correlation between electro-echocardiographic parameters and cirrhosis severity scores (CHILD PUGH and MELD)

Parameters		CHILD PUGH	MELD
DOG	r	0,189	0,225
	p	0,108	0,054
VOG	r	**0,351**	**0,329**
	p	**0,002**	**0,004**
VTD	r	-0,106	-0,087
	p	0,368	0,460
VTS	r	-0,068	-0,093
	p	0,565	0,431
DTD	r	0,095	0,024
	p	0,419	0,838
DTS	r	0,084	0,002
	p	0,474	0,984

SIV	r	0,038	0,045
	p	0,742	0,702
PPVG	r	0,118	0,143
	p	0,309	0,218
LVEF	r	0,008	0,203
	p	0,943	0,078
SLG	r	0,058	0,184
	p	0,623	0,116
E/A	r	0,11	0,079
	p	0,347	0,502
TRIV	r	-0,102	-0,107
	p	0,388	0,365
TDE	r	0,27	0,83
	p	0,82	0,47
E/E'	r	0,033	0,06
	p	0,77	0,96

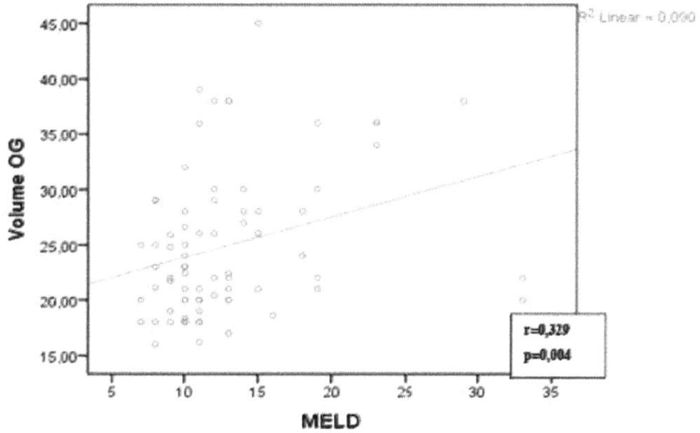

Figure 18: Correlation between MELD score and left atrial volume

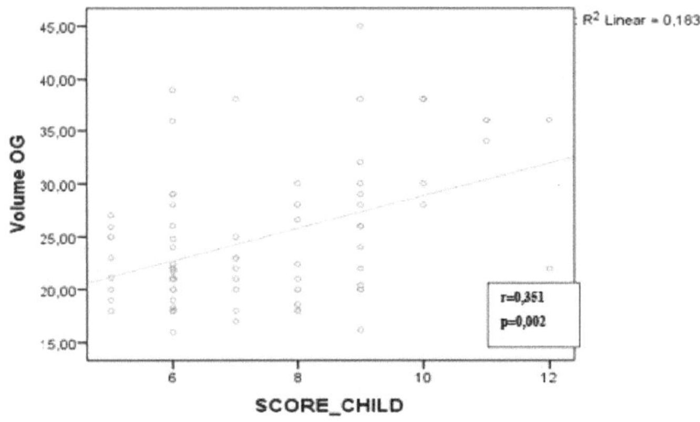

Figure 19: Correlation between CHILD PUGH score and left atrial volume

> There was also a statistically significant positive correlation between the QT interval and the two cirrhosis sëvëritë scores (Table XIV): MELD.*(Figure20)and* CHILD PUGH *(Figure 21).*

Table XIV: Correlation between QT interval and cirrhosis severity scores
(CHILD PUGH and MELD)

Parameters		CHILD PUGH	MELD
QT interval	r	0,292	0,329
	P	0,011	0,004

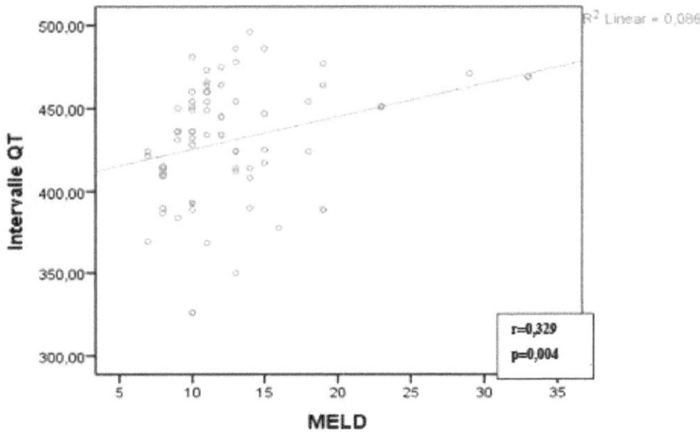

Figure 20: Correlation between MELD score and QT interval

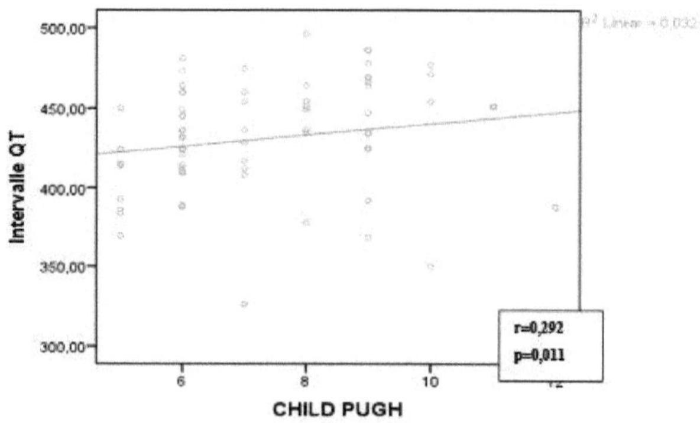

Figure 21: Correlation between CHILD PUGH score and QT interval

4 DISCUSSION

Despite all the attention paid to hëmodynamic disturbances during cirrhosis, the heart itself was relatively ignored (4). It was not until the 1980s that successive experimental and clinical ëtudies confirmed the presence of cardiac dysfunction Hë to cirrhosis, independent of its ëtiology, baptisedë "cirrhotic cardiomyopathy" (1,24).

Starting out as a simple scientific curiosity, CMC has evolved into a clinical entity in its own right, which has aroused undeniable interest in recent years, due to its impact on the management of cirrhotic patients (6).

In everyday practice, cardiac abnormalities in cirrhotic patients are not systematically investigated in our country.

In this study, we set out to determine the prevalence of CMC in patients treated for cirrhosis in the hepato-gastro-enterology department of the Sahloul University Hospital in Sousse, and to identify its predictive factors. We also studied the correlation between electrochocardiographic parameters and the severity of liver disease. Finally, we assessed the contribution of new echocardiographic techniques in the positive diagnosis of this entity.

To this end, we conducted a cross-sectional study of 76 cirrhotic patients. Patients with cardiovascular comorbidities or conditions that could affect cardiac function, such as sëvëre anemia or recent digestive bleeding, were not included. On the one hand, this choice made it possible to link the electro- echocardiographic abnormalities to the underlying hepatic disease but, on the other hand, limited the number of patients in the study.

The mean age of the patients was 54 years. Cirrhosis was of viral origin in 35 cases (46%). It was classified as CHILD PUGH B in 34 patients (44.7%). The median MELD score was 11. Our population benefited from a clinical examination, an ECG and a TTE: conventional, tissue Doppler, as well as a 2D Strain study.

1. PHYSIOPATHOLOGICAL BASES :

The pathophysiology of cirrhotic cardiomyopathy is multifactorial *(Figure 22)*. It is associated with :

1.1. DYSFUNCTION OF THE B-ADRENERGIC PATHWAY :

Myocyte contractility is governed primarily by b-adrenergic stimulation which, following a cascade of intracellular signals, leads to binding between 1 actin and myosin, resulting in cell contraction(25) . The abnormalities dëcribed in the cirrhotic patient that impair contractile function dë begin at the level of these signals and propagate to downstream transduction pathways (26-30). Numerous ëstudies have demonstrated a decrease in b-adrenergic receptor density and sensitivity in cardiomyocytes.

1.2. DYSFUNCTION OF THE CARDIOINHIBITORY SYSTEMS:

Cardioinhibitory systëmes are mainly regulated by endocannabinoi'des, TNF-a, NO (nitric oxide) and CO (carbon monoxide) (31-36). Endocannabinoids exert a negative inotropic effect on the heart and are stimulated in cirrhosis. NO and CO are inert gases produced in the heart via the enzymes NO-synthase and hëme-oxygënase-1 respectively; both stimulate the production of cyclic guanosine monophosphate (cGMP) which induces inhibition of intracellular calcium flow and hence contractile response. These two enzymes are strongly induced in cirrhosis and therefore contribute to the cardiodepressor effect.

1.3. STRUCTURAL ABNORMALITIES OF CARDIOMYOCYTES :

Experimental studies have shown an increase in the cholesterol/phospholipid ratio and membrane rigidity in cardiomyocytes from cirrhotic rats (37). This alteration in membrane fluidity leads to an alteration in the function of ion channels such as the calcium-independent potassium channel (25,38-41). Among other things, this results in a prolongation of the action potential and therefore of the QT interval (42,43).

1.4. ROLE OF BILE ACIDS :

Defects in the regulation of bile acid metabolism have been shown to play an important role in the development of myocardial dysfunction (44,45).

Rë Recently, Desai et al foundë, in an experimental model, that the ëchographic earaeteristics of cardiomyopathy resolved after normalisation of bile acid serum levels (46). These results argue for a direct and reversible effect of bile acids on cardiomyocytes.

1.5. ROLE OF HEMODYNAMIC ABNORMALITIES IN CIRRHOSIS:

Persistent hyperdynamic circulation with increased cardiac output and frequency plays a role in myocardial hypertrophy (47). In addition, prolonged activation of the renin-angiotensin-aldosterone system may also be involved, inducing fibrosis in the heart (45,48-50). Fluid retention can also lead to the generation of edema, not only in the form of ascites and peripheral edema but also in the myocardium(30,51).

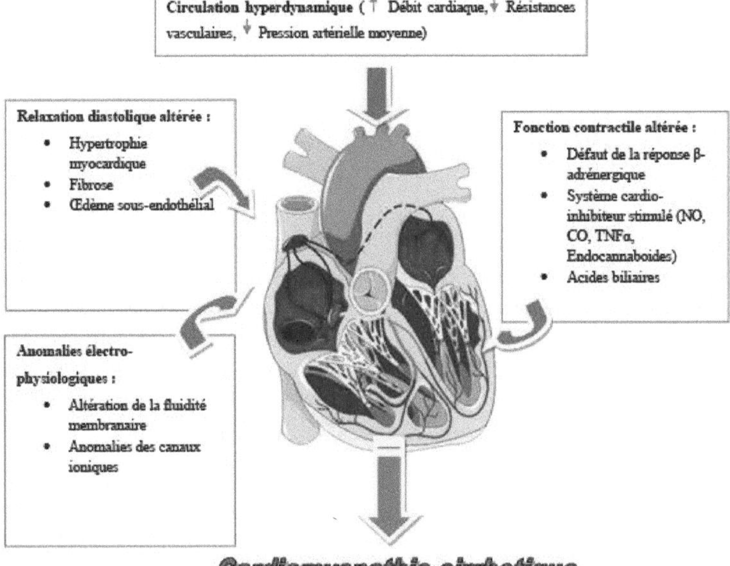

Hyperdynamic circulation (cardiac output, vascular resistance, mean arterial pressure)
Impaired diastolic relaxation :
"Myocardial hypertrophy " Fibrosis " Subendothelial oedema
Electro-physiological abnormalities :

"Impaired membrane fluidity " Ion channel abnormalities
Impaired contractile function :
"Defective β-adrenergic response Stimulated cardioinhibitory system (NO, CO, TNFα, endocannabinoids) Bile acids

Figure 22: Schematic representation of the anomalies associated with the pathophysiology of cirrhotic cardiomyopathy

2. DEFINITION AND PREVALENCE OF CIRRHOTIC CARDIOMYOPATHY :

CMC is the term used to designate all abnormalities of cardiac structure and function in cirrhotics. It appears to be inseparable from the hypercinetic syndrome and would fall within the framework of heart failure with a ëleyë rate (52).

Specific diagnostic criteria for CMC were formulated by a consensus committee of hepatologists and cardiologists at the WCG in 2005, including :

Systolic dysfunction, defined as:

> Alteration of cardiac output in response to exercise, changes in vascular volume and pharmacological stimuli.

> Ejection fraction < 55% at rest

Diastolic dysfunction, defined by:

> E/A<1

> Extended deceleration time (> 200ms)

> Prolongation of iso-volumetric time (> 80ms)

Support criteria :

> Electrophysiological abnormalities including: altered chronotropic response to stress, electromechanical decoupling, QTc prolongation

> Dilatation of the left atrium

> Increase in myocardial mass

> Elevation of BNP or Nt-Pro BNP

> Elevation of troponin I

Using this definition, the prevalence of CMC in our series was 53.9%.

The exact prevalence of CMC is difficult to determine. This is partly due to the fact that CMC often remains a latent phenomenon, difficult to recognise clinically apart from a stress stimulus (3,53-55). In addition, the current consensus definition seems inadequate and open to discussion due to its lack of precision. The minimum number of criteria required for diagnosis and the relevance of each criterion (major or minor) have not been specified.

Also, the majority of ëtudies published in the literature have focusedëes on one of the three major abnormalities that characterise MCC, namely: DS, DD, or electrophysiological abnormalities leading in particular to QT interval prolongation.

2.1. SYSTOLIC DYSFUNCTION :

Assessment of systolic function according to the WCG 2005 consensus is based on LVEF, with SD defined as LVEF<55%. Based on this definition, the prevalence of resting SD in cirrhotic patients was low in different studies, ranging from 0 to 10%, which is in agreement with the results of our series, where SD was found in 5.3% of patients *(Table XV)*.

Table XV: Prevalence of systolic dysfunction in cirrhotic patients in the literature

	Number of patients	Systolic dysfunction (%)
Sampaio et al 2013(56)	109	9,2
Nazar et al 2013(57)	152	0
Merli et al 2013(58)	74	0
Sampaio et al 2014(59)	98	10,2
Carvalheiro et al. 2016(55)	106	1,1
Devi et al 2017(60)	60	10
Our study	76	5,3%

This low prevalence may be explained by the dependence of LVEF on loading conditions, and it is well established that cirrhotic patients have a decrease in afterload due to reduced peripheral vascular resistance(56,61-64). Thus, a normal LVEF at rest cannot reflect normal contractility. This underlines the value of stress testing in investigating systolic function in cirrhotic patients(53,65). In the literature, few studies have assessed systolic function using stress tests. Sampaio et al, in a case-control study published in 2015, studied systolic function in 36 cirrhotic patients using stress cardiac MRI under dobutamine (66). The authors concluded that patients with cirrhosis show, in the face of pharmacological stress, an incompëtence inotropic due to intrinseal myocardial dysfunction. This result was ëlë repeated in a ëtude by Kim et al. or a ëstress echocardiography under dobutamine ëloк performed in 71 cirrhotics with a normal LVEF at rest, a DS (ckf'inie by an increase of less than 10% in LVEF) ëloк observed in 25.4% of cases(67). Rë recently also, Barbosa et al. suggestedërë that stress lkchocardiography under dobutamine is an important tool for the diagnosis of CMC. However, to date, no stress test has ële validatedë for 1 exploration of cardiac function in cirrhotic patients.

2.2. DIASTOLIC DYSFUNCTION :

Over the last two dëcennies, several ëtudes have intëressëes to ëevaluate diastolic function in cirrhotics. The majority of them showed that the E/A ratio ëloк significantly lower and that TDE and TRIV ëtaient significativement plus ëlevës chez les cirrhotiques par rapport aux tëmoins (68-70). These three parameters were used in the consensus definition of CMC to define DD. In our sërie, more than пюШё of patients (51.4%) had DD according to these diagnostic criteria. Our results concur with those of the literature since most of the public sëries report prevalences ëlevëes varying between 30 and 67%.*(Table XVI)*

Table XVI: Prevalences of diastolic dysfunction (on conventional echocardiography) in cirrhotic patients in the literature

	Number of patients	Diastolic dysfunction(%)
Sampanio et al. 2013(56)	109	40,4
Nazar et al. 2013(57)	102	58

Alexopoulou et al. 2012(71)	76	67
Papastergiou et al. 2012(72)	92	59,8
Chen et al. 2016(73)	103	44
Devi et al 2017(60)	60	31,6
Our study	76	51,4

2.3. ELECTROCARDIOGRAPHIC ABNORMALITIES:

Three main abnormalities are described during cirrhosis: prolongation of the QT interval, chronotropic incompetence and ëlectromëcanic dëcoupling.(24) Prolongation of the QT interval is the most frequent ëlëctrocardiographic abnormality (74).

The QT interval in fact refutes ëlectromëcanic synchronisation: dëlai between the ëlectrical excitation phase and ^xëв^шм mëcanic. Its duration varies inversely with heart rate, so correct interpretation of the QT interval requires a correction in relation to it. This can be done using various formulae, of which the "QTc cirrhosis" formula would be the most appropriate for cirrhotic patients because of a QT-RR indëpendence coefficient close to 0(28,75,76). Adopting this formula, we found that 43.5% of cirrhotic patients had QTc prolongation. These results are comparable to those found in the literature, where the prevalence varies from 24 to 65%. (*Table XVII*).

Table XVII: Prevalences of QTc prolongation in cirrhotic patients
in the literature

Studies	Number of patients	Prolongation [QT] (%)
Hansen et *al. 2007* (77)	23	47
Li et *al.* 2007 (78)	126	47
Genovesi et *al.* 2008 (79)	48	64,5
Bhatti et *al.* 2014 (80)	166	24,6
Kim et *al.* *2017* (81)	406	51
Our study	76	43,5

2.4. OTHER ABNORMALITIES ASSOCIATED WITH CARDIOMYOPATHY CIRRHOTIC :

2.4.1. Morphological changes in the heart cavities :

In addition to the above abnormalities, MCC is characterised by a number of morphological changes in the heart. These changes appear to affect mainly the left cavities and may include both volume and pressure abnormalities, as well as myocardial mass. In the 2005 consensus definition of MCC, only increased myocardial mass and left atrial dilatation are included as supporting criteria.

The size of the left atrium is at the crossroads of cardiovascular pathophysiology and is a powerful prognostic marker in multiple pathologies (82,83). VOG, from prëfërence indexë to body surface area, is an important measure for re-evaluating diastolic function. This parameter is considered to reflect the severity and age of the volume and/or pressure overload imposed on the atrium(83). In our study, 59.2% of patients had left atrial dilatation as evidenced by an indexed VOG>34 ml/m2. Furthermore, when correlating different echocardiographic parameters with cirrhosis severity scores, VOG was the only parameter with a significant positive correlation with both the CHILD PUGH score and the MELD score (r=0.329 and r= 0.351 respectively). Our results are in line with those published in the literature. Indeed, the increase in left atrial volume is well documented and appears to be related to advanced liver disease as reported by some authors (47,68). Finucci et al. assessed diastolic function in 42 cirrhotics and 16 controls by Doppler echocardiography (84). Compared with the control group, patients had a significantly higher indexed VOG (31 ± 10 mL / m^2 vs 20 ± 7 mL / m^2 , p <0.0001). The positive correlation of VOG with MELD score was also found in the study by Li et al ($r = 0.208;P < 0.05$) (85). Furthermore, in the study by Ruiz-Del-Arbol et al, cirrhotic patients with DD had a significantly higher indexed VOG than those with normal diastolic function (5). The authors also concluded that indexed VOG was predictive of survival at 12 months. This finding was confirmed by a recent study published in 2016 with a 24-month follow-up (86).

These results suggest that OG dilatation, while considered a secondary criterion defining CMC, should be adopted as a primary marker of this entity, the presence of which would be associated with advanced and decompensated cirrhosis, and would make it possible to identify patients at risk of developing cardiac dysfunction.

In addition, several clinical and autopsy studies have reported the presence of LVH in cirrhotic patients (87-89). This anomaly was present in 15.8% of our patients. In the study by Yan Chen et al. including 103 patients with cirrhosis, left ventricular mass was higher in cirrhotic patients than in controls ($208.5 \pm$ 57.5 vs 175.6 ± 42.8 g; p<0.01) (90). This study was the first to prospectively demonstrate that in patients with cirrhosis awaiting liver transplantation, there is a significant progressive increase in left ventricular thickness and mass.

2.4.2. Seric markers :

There are a number of serum markers that are routinely used in the diagnosis, monitoring and prognosis of heart failure(91). Among these markers, BNP (brain natriuretic peptide) and its precursor NT pro-BNP, as well as Troponin I, are the most widely studied in patients with cirrhosis(92). Plasma BNP levels are thought to correlate with the severity of liver disease and its cardiac repercussions (their levels are proportional to QT interval prolongation, SIV thickening and DTS) (93-95). Similarly, troponin I levels may be increased, but less consistently (96). These results indicate the potential usefulness of these serum markers for diagnosing myocardial distress in cirrhosis, but specific criteria such as exact diagnostic threshold values remain to be determined.

Many other proteins with enzymatic activity, such as myeloperoxidase, galectin-3 and copeptin, have been linked to cardiac damage in cirrhosis, but the results of studies remain controversial (97,98).

3. NEW TECHNOLOGIES

ECHOCARDIOGRAPHY IN THE DIAGNOSIS OF CIRRHOTIC CARDIOMYOPATHY :

3.1. STRAIN SPECKLE TRACKING OR TWO-DIMENSIONAL STRAIN (STRAIN 2D) :

Strain 2D is an innovative echocardiographic technique. It allows analysis of myocardial deformation in three orthogonal directions: longitudinal,
circumferential and radial.

Based on the recording of a two-dimensional echocardiographic loop, Strain 2D makes it possible to track the various acoustic speckles contained in a region of the myocardial wall throughout the cardiac cycle and to analyse their displacement relative to one another. In this way, we can obtain the segmental or global strain of the left ventricle in different directions: the longitudinal strain obtained on apical sections, the radial strain, and the circumferential strain obtained on parasternal sections.

Alteration of longitudinal strain is more precocious than that of radial or circumferential strain in subclinical heart disease and suggests subendocardial involvement. Longitudinal strain is also the most reproducible with a coefficient of variation around 6% (99). In our work, we intéressés to study this paramëtre which defines systolic dysfunction by a value <-18%.

The clinical applications of this technique, which is simple and reproducible, are increasing in number and encompass ever wider areas (100-102). It has been validated and recommended as a diagnostic and prognostic tool in valvulopathies and in hypertrophic, ischemic and radio-chemo-induced cardiomyopathies (103).

Although its role in the diagnosis of cardiomyopathy in cirrhotics remains unclear, a few recent studies have suggested its usefulness in demonstrating myocardial dysfunction in this population (6,7,104). Using this technique, Simpaio et al. demonstrated the presence of altered left ventricular longitudinal strain in cirrhotics compared with controls, suggesting subendocardial dysfunction (105). A more recent study demonstrated the presence, in cirrhotic patients with normal FEVG, of an alteration of the
Strain of the left ventricle in the three orthogonal directions, indicating transmural myocardial damage (73).

In our series, 10 patients (13%) had an LMS value < -18%, 6 of whom had a normal LVEF.

These results show that this technique can be useful for early detection of alteration in left ventricular systolic function even before the LOS defined by calculation of LVEF occurs.

3.2. TISSUE DOPPLER :

It is currently well established that diastolic vëlocitës measured by tissue Doppler across the mitral annulus play a major role in Evaluation of DD. Indeed, the recommendations for Evaluation of left ventricular diastolic function were updated in 2009(106) and then most recently in 2016   (107). The four variables

Recommendations for identifying a DD are: peak early diastolic vëlocitë (E '), E/E' ratio, indexed left atrial volume and maximum tricuspid insufficiency velocity.

Although the diagnostic work-up for DD is clearly advancedë, the use of these new mëthods in cirrhosis has been limited to a few ëtudes. Using this diagnostic approach, the prevalence of DD in 109 cirrhotics in the study by Sampaio et al. was 16.5%. In the same study, the prevalence of DD based on the 2005 consensus definition was 40.4%. These results are in agreement with those of our study, since the prevalence of DD based on tissue Doppler data was lower than that defined by conventional parameters (39.2% vs 51.3%).

Echocardiography coupled with tissue Doppler provides a more adequate assessment of diastolic function than that based on transmitral flow (108-111). Variations in pre-load and heart rate can significantly alter the E/A ratio and EDT, even in normal subjects (112). This can be a major problem in cirrhotic patients, as they usually have a lower pre-load and often a higher HR, resulting in a lower E/A ratio regardless of the presence or absence of a relaxation disorder (113). On the other hand, the E' wave represents a sensitive marker of myocardial relaxation disorder, being independent of load conditions(107). The E/E' ratio also allows adequate estimation of ventricular filling pressures (107).

However, the use of the new recommendations has proved more complex, leading to a certain variability in the assessment of DD, even among expert echocardiographers. This probably explains some of the differences in the prevalence of DD among the most recent studies in cirrhosis *(Table XVIII)*.

Table XVIII: Prevalences of diastolic dysfunction (according to the new recommendations) in cirrhotic patients in the literature

	Number of patients	Diastolic dysfunction(%)
Sampanio et al. 2014(105)	98	16,3
Somani et al. 2014(114)	60	30
Karagiannakis et al. 2013(115)	44	37,8
Ruiz et al. 2013(16)	80	46,2
Falletta et al. 2015(116)	84	26
Rimbas et al. 2017(117)	46	47,8
Our study	76	32,9

3.3. PREVALENCE OF CIRRHOTIC CARDIOMYOPATHY USING NEW ECHOCARDIOGRAPHIC TECHNIQUES:

Based on data from the new ëchocardiographic modalities, the prevalence of CMC in our series was lower compared with that retained on conventional criteria (40.8% vs 53.9%) with moderate agreement between the two definitions (kappa index equal to 0.585). Similar results have been reported in recently published studies, the conclusions of which suggest the integration of these new parameters in the assessment of cardiac function in cirrhosis, as they are both more sensitive and more specific than conventional parameters(90,105,117). In view of the particular hemodynamic characteristics of cirrhotic patients, and taking into account the often silent nature of this cardiac dysfunction, tissue Doppler and 2D Strain would provide a more appropriate approach to this entity. The diagnostic criteria for CMC therefore need to be updated and subsequently validated in large-scale prospective studies.

4. FACTORS PREDICTIVE OF CIRRHOTIC CARDIOMYOPATHY :

In our study, univariate analysis of the various demographic, clinical, biological and ëlëctro-ëchocardiographic parameters revealed that age, female sex, CHILD PUGH score>9 and moderate to severe renal insufficiency (creatinine clearance<60ml/min) were factors associated with CMC.

Multivariate analysis identified 3 independent predictors of MCC: age (OR 1.05; 95% CI :1.003-1.103; p<0.039), female sex (OR 3.006; CI95%: 1.029-8.778; p=0.044) and CHILD PUGH score>9 (OR 4.363; CI95%: 1.328-14.331; p=0.015).

In the literature, not many studies have sought to identify factors predictive of CMC. In the study by Belay et al. published in 2013, CMC was diagnosed in 51% of the 231 cirrhotic patients included. Patients with CMC were significantly older (62.7 vs 57.8 years; p < 0.001) and more female than male (55.8 vs 40.2%; p = 0.02). In multivariate analysis, age was the only independent predictor of CMC (OR 1.6; IC95%:1.2 - 2; p<0.001). This is consistent with the findings of a second study published in the same year, involving 45 cirrhotics, where age was also found to be an independent predictor of CMC (OR 1.081; 95% CI 1.007-1.159; p= 0.031). Papastergiou et al. concluded in their prospective study, which included 92 cirrhotics, that age > 53 years was also a predictive factor for CMC with an OR of 4.2 (95% CI: 1.5-12.1) (72).

The majority of studies, including our own, agree that CMC is independent of the etiology of cirrhosis (72,118).

The link between CMC and the severity of cirrhosis remains controversial, with sometimes contradictory results. In our study, the CHILD PUGH score >9 had the highest predictive value, with an OR of 4.363 (IC95%:1.328-14.331). However, there was no association between MELD score and CMC. This is in agreement with the study by Papastergiou et al, where CHILD PUGH stage C was an independent predictor of CMC with an OR of 4.6 (CI95%:1.1-20)(72). In contrast, Merli et al showed that the presence of ascites was significantly associated with DD (p=0.04) (58). However, neither the CHILD PUGH score nor the MELD score was predictive of cardiac dysfunction. Indeed, the different ëchocardiographic ëparameters were comparable between the CHILD PUGH B/C vs CHILD PUGH A patient groups and MELD<15 vs MELD>15.

Pozzi et al. in their prospective study aimed at assessing cardiac function in patients with chronic viral C hepatopathy, concluded that there was no association between DD and the CHILD PUGH score (118) .

5. IMPLICATIONS OF CARDIOMYOPATHY CIRRHOTICS :

5.1. INVOLVEMENT IN THE GENESIS OF HEPATO-RENAL SYNDROME:

HRS is a functional renal failure complicating decompensated cirrhosis(119). From a pathophysiological point of view, systemic arterial vasodilatation appears to be at the forefront (120). In order to maintain arterial pressure, stimulation of the renin-angiotensin-aldosterone system ensues, leading to arterial vasoconstriction, particularly of the renal vascular bed. Recent studies suggest that CMC contributes to the development of SHR through altered cardiac contractility and reduced cardiac output, which exacerbate renal hypoperfusion (16,52,65,121).

Ruiz-Del-Arbol et al. showed that patients with cirrhosis who developed HRS during spontaneous ascites fluid infection had significantly lower cardiac output than those who maintained normal renal function (5.7 ± 0.9 vs. 7.4 ± 1.9 L/min)(122). Moreover, even after resolution of the infection, patients with renal insufficiency maintained an even lower cardiac output (4.6 ± 0.7 vs. 6.8 ± 2.0 L/min). Later, the same team carried out a second prospective study in 66 patients with cirrhosis complicated by refractory ascites, 40% of whom had developed SHR (52). The authors showed that patients who developed SHR had a lower baseline cardiac output than those who did not (6.0 ± 1.2 vs. 7.2 ± 1.8 l/min). In this study, increased plasma renin activity and low cardiac output proved to be powerful determinants in the development of SHR. Thus, the inability of the heart to maintain normal contractility, which defines, among other things, CMC, as well as the worsening of peripheral vasodilatation, appear to be of major importance in the development of renal dysfunction and HRS.

Krag et al. also demonstrated a significant relationship between the degree of systolic dysfunction and renal function in patients with decompensated cirrhosis (123).

Finally, it emerges from these results that, during cirrhosis, there appears to be a complex, bidirectional relationship between the heart and kidneys, which has тёпе suggested to us that we should refine the definition of SHR in order to recognise the symbiotic link between these two organs.

By applying this theoretical knowledge, a Brazilian team recently pioneered the treatment of type 1 SHR refractory to conventional therapies in patients with cirrhosis and a clinical diagnosis of CCM, in whom the use of dobutamine as rescue therapy was successful (124).

In our series, patients with CMC had lower creatinine clearance compared with those with normal cardiac function. Very intëressingly, we also notedë, that in univariate analysis, the presence of moderate to severe renal failure (defined as clearance <60ml/min/d) was significantly associated with CMC (p=0.004).

Given that patients with MCC are likely to develop HRS, especially if an acute event (in particular an ascites fluid infection) disrupts their precarious circulatory state, particular vigilance should be exercised in this group of patients in order to anticipate this formidable complication.

5.2. THERAPEUTIC IMPLICATIONS :

5.2.1. If medical treatment is started :

Heart failure may occur in the event of sudden variations in cardiac load conditions. Thus, massive infusions of albumin, as for example during an ascites fluid infection where the prescription of albumin at an initial dose of 1.5g/kg followed by a dose of 1g/kg on the third day is indicated, may cause pulmonary redëme by abruptly increasing preload.

CMC may also occur in the event of a direct reduction in myocardial contractility, particularly when beta-blocker therapy is introduced too rapidly(125).

Cirrhotic patients often require dose adjustment when prescribing mëdicaments. There is a close correlation between prognostic scores (MELD and Child-Pugh) and drug clearance(126). Also, cytochrome P450 3A activity is reduced in cirrhotics(127). Consequently, the prescription of QT-prolonging drugs in cirrhotics may be potentially dangerous. Some of these drugs, such as quinolones and vasopressin, are commonly used in cirrhosis and others are sometimes prescribed, such as amiodarone and macrolides. However, it is not yet known whether their prescription in cirrhotic patients entails an increased risk of ventricular arrhythmia compared with non-cirrhotic patients. In this respect, a case of torsade de pointes in a cirrhotic woman during amiodarone infusion for arrhythmia due to atrial fibrillation was recently described (128). Werner et *al.* reported a case of torsade de pointes in a cirrhotic treated with quinolones and hemopressin for variceal haemorrhage (129). Lehmann et al. described the case of a cirrhotic who required cardio-respiratory resuscitation after an infusion of terlipressin(130). For quinolones, the arrhythmogenic potential varies from one molecule to another, being greater with moxifloxacin than with ciprofloxacin and norfloxacin, which are the molecules most commonly used in cirrhotics(131). As a consequence, many drugs potentially affecting ventricular repolarisation are rather inconsiderately used in daily practice. Given this context, caution is advised when administering the above-mentioned drugs in cirrhotic patients (132).

5.2.2. If a trans-jugular intra-hepatic porto-systemic shunt (TIPS) is inserted:

The introduction of a TIPS is also associated with a sudden increase in preload, which can even double the cardiac output. This diversion of portal flow into the systemic venous circulation can therefore have major hemodynamic repercussions on the heart of a cirrhotic. Some studies have shown that post-TIPS cardiac decompensation occurs in 12% to 13% of patients. Cazzaniga and colleagues demonstrated that echocardiographic measurement of the E/A ratio 4 weeks after insertion of the TIPS was the only independent predictor of survival following this procedure (133). It should therefore be remembered that this procedure represents considerable hëmodynamic stress and may dëmasquer latent cardiomyopathy in cirrhotic patients. It is therefore advisable to carry out cardiological investigations (ECG, echocardiography) in search of CMC before considering TIPS.

5.2.3. In the event of liver transplantation:

Liver transplantation represents the most severe clinical situation, in terms of cardiovascular stress, that a cirrhotic patient may encounter. Indeed, an increase in both preload and afterload is observed in the perioperative period. The cirrhotic patient may be unable to manage these changes, revealing underlying myocardial dysfunction(125).

Mittal et al. followed 970 cirrhotic liver transplant recipients over a mean period of 5.3 years and found that pre-transplant DD significantly increased the risk of graft rejection and mortality. The authors emphasised the importance of cardiac evaluation during the pre-transplant period (134).

This is consistent with the findings of Dowsley et al. who found that markers of DD, namely E/E'>10 and index VOG >40 mL/m2 on preoperative TTE, increased the risk of heart failure after liver transplantation by 3.4-fold and 2.9-fold respectively (135).

Currently, heart failure following liver transplantation is recognised as a distinct clinical entity, associated with high mortality, and occurs in the absence of any obvious risk factors (136). It is the third leading cause of intraoperative mortality (7-21%) in this setting, after graft rejection and infectious complications (3,137,138). However, to date, there are no reliable tests to identify patients at risk of developing this complication. In light of these data, the American Society of Liver Transplantation recently published (in January 2018) new recommendations aimed at identifying recipients at risk of developing heart failure (54). These recommendations highlighted the importance of a precise and complete pre-transplant cardiac evaluation, including a 12-lead ECG, TTE and stress echocardiography if signs suggestive of latent DS are present.

5.3. PROGNOSTIC IMPLICATIONS :

The association between CMC and prognosis remains controversial, with hëtërogënes reported in different studies (Table XIX).

In their prospective study with a 12-month follow-up, Somani et al. found that there was no significant difference between the survival of cirrhotic patients with normal diastolic function and those with DD (139).

On the other hand, Karagiannakis et al. concluded, in a prospective study including 45 patients with cirrhosis of different etiologies, that DD and hypoalbuminemia were the only independent predictive factors of mortality after a follow-up of 24 months (115). Also, in the series by Ruiz et al, the E/E' ratio was found to be an independent predictor of mortality (16). In the same study, survival was found to be correlated with the severity of DD. One-year survival was significantly higher in patients with normal diastolic function (95%) compared with those with grade 1 (79%) or grade 2 (39%) DD (16).

In addition, several authors suggest that QT interval prolongation in cirrhotic patients is associated with a poorer prognosis. Bernardi et al. found that the survival of cirrhotics with prolonged QT was shorter than that of cirrhotics with normal QT(140). Also, in the recent study by Kim et al, the QT interval was an independent predictor of mortality (OR 1.69, 95%CI: 1.032.77, P= 0.039) (81).

Also, in the context of upper gastrointestinal haemorrhage, Trevisiani et al found two independent factors predictive of mortality: the MELD score and the duration of the QT interval(14).

Table XIX: Studies evaluating the prognostic role of cardiac parameters in cirrhotic patients

Studies	Number of patients	Duration of follow-up (months)	Prognostic parameters
Krag et al(123)	24	12	- Cardiac index<1.5l/min/m2
Merli et al(86)	90	24	- increase in the size of the OG - reduced LV mass
Ruiz-Del-Arbol et	80	12	- increase in the E/E' ratio

al(16)			-DD	
Cesari et al(141)	115	72	-	increase in the size of the OG
			-	increase in the E/E' ratio
			-	increase in Fc
			-	reduction in MAP

6. THERAPEUTIC MANAGEMENT OF CIRRHOTIC CARDIOMYOPATHY:

The specific management of MCC currently remains unclear. Furthermore, there are very few studies in humans on the treatment of manifestations of this entity (142,143). Fortunately, in the absence of coexisting alcoholic cardiomyopathy, severe overt heart failure remains rare.

Nevertheless, if this complication occurs, the same general principles of treatment for non-cirrhotic heart failure apply, with one important caveat: afterload reduction, a mainstay of heart failure treatment in non-cirrhotic patients, must be done with caution in patients with cirrhosis. The majority of these patients already have arterial hypotension, and the aggressive administration of vasodilators may precipitate the collapse of effective blood flow, leading to renal dysfunction.

Theoretically, pharmacological agents that improve cardiac compliance and LV relaxation would be the ideal treatment for DD. Thus, в-blockers, calcium channel blockers, ACE inhibitors and angiotensin II receptor blockers (ARBs) are the molecules most commonly used in patients with DD.

ACE inhibitors and ARB IIs are probably effective in slowing the progression of grade 1 DD. However, these molecules are contraindicated in cirrhotic patients because they can induce functional renal failure by inhibiting the vasoconstrictive effect of Angiotensin II on the efferent arteriole of the renal glomerulus.

The в-blockers, long known for their effect on portal hypertension and prevention of rupture of esophageal varices, appear to have a more favourable benefit/risk profile. An improvement in cardiac function has been observed by shortening the QTc interval (144). However, в-blockers are ineffective in grade II DD. Indeed, experimental animal studies have demonstrated an alteration in protodiastolic relaxation by в-blockers (145). In addition, в-blockers may be impaired by a reduction in cardiac output. Thus, their prescription is associated with a guarded prognosis in cases of refractory ascites (146).

Another class of very promising médicaments in this pathology are the aldostěrone antagonists, which have shown a significant běněйce on ventricular wall remodelling and diastolic function, without having the nebitic hěmodynamic and renal effect observed with ACE inhibitors (147). Indeed, Pozzi et al. showed a change in left ventricular cavity dimensions and a decrease in myocardial wall thickness after 6 months of treatment with anti-aldosterone (148). A slight but not significant improvement in diastolic function was noted, which is why the authors suggested extending the duration of treatment.

Liver transplantation remains the ultimate curative treatment for cirrhosis and virtually all its complications, including cardiac dysfunction. Indeed, it appears that liver transplantation leads to an improvement in the main aspects of CMC within 6 to 9 months post-transplant(149). However, the peri-operative phase remains critical, particularly in view of the various hemodynamic complications that may arise (150).

7. LIMITS OF THE STUDY:

The limitations of our study were :

> Its cross-sectional nature means that we are unable to follow the development of electrocardiographic abnormalities over time, their impact on the survival curve, and above all to investigate whether assessment of cardiac function using the new echocardiographic techniques can be a relevant prognostic marker.

> Furthermore, our study did not include serum markers, in particular ProBNP, recognised as an important marker in the evaluation of diastolic function, or a stress test (physical activity or pharmacological stress) which could have better revealed latent cardiac dysfunction.

> It should also be noted that cirrhotic patients may concomitantly present with secondary cardiac damage such as ischemic heart disease; a ëventualitë that has not been formally ëliminatedëe.

8. RECOMMENDATIONS :

At the end of this work, we recommend the following measures:

✓ It is vital to better define the diagnostic criteria for CMC, and to update the ëchocardiographic criteria by including tissue Doppler and Strain2D parameters. Indeed, re-evaluating cardiac function by measuring conventional parameters alone now seems anachronistic in the light of the new techniques available.

✓ This silent entity should be systematically investigated in cirrhotic patients, given its frequency, its presence at different stages of liver disease, and its major importance in the management of these patients. This would make it possible to:

✓ avoid untimely treatments that could mask cardiac dysfunction, in particular massive albumin infusions or beta-blocker treatment started rapidly at full dose.

✓ to anticipate a deterioration in renal function and possibly a SHR, particularly in the event of an intercurrent event such as an infection or digestive haemorrhage, by monitoring the renal balance and ensuring adequate vascular filling.

✓ to selectively improve cardiac function when necessary and possible, particularly prior to surgery or TIPS.

5 CONCLUSION

Cirrhotic cardiomyopathy" (CMC), a relatively recent and long-neglected concept, is currently emerging as a specific clinical entity, characterised by systolic dysfunction (SD), diastolic dysfunction (DD) and electrophysiological abnormalities, occurring in cirrhotic patients in the absence of any known cardiac pathology. Its diagnosis is essentially based on echocardiography, whose recent advances, culminating in tissue Doppler and 2D Strain, have led to a paradigm shift in the analysis of cardiac function.

In this context, we conducted a cross-sectional analytical study in the cniepiito-giistroenteroiogy department of the Sahloul University Hospital in Sousse, over a period of 9 months. The aim of our study was to determine the prevalence of CMC and to investigate its predictive factors. In addition, we studied the correlation between echocardiographic parameters and the severity of liver disease. We also assessed the contribution of new cardiac ultrasound techniques to the positive diagnosis of this condition.

Our study population included 76 cirrhotic patients. Cirrhosis was confirmed histologically or based on a combination of clinical, biological, endoscopic and morphological evidence, including signs of hepatocellular failure and portal hypertension. Patients with a history of cardiovascular disease, obesity, chronic alcoholism or other conditions that could affect cardiac function (such as severe anaemia or recent digestive haemorrhage) were not included in the study. Each patient in our population benefited from a clinical examination, a biological work-up, an ECG to calculate the QT interval and cardiac ultrasound in two-dimensional mode, tissue Doppler and 2D Strain.

The patients were divided into 45 men (59% of patients) and 31 women (41%). Their average age was 54, with extremes ranging from 18 to 79 years. In the majority of cases (46%), cirrhosis was of viral origin: post-viral B cirrhosis in 30 patients (39.5%) and post-viral C cirrhosis in 5 patients (6.6%). She was classified as CHILD PUGH B in 45% of cases. The CHILD PUGH score was >9 in 30.3% of patients. The MELD score was >15 in 22.4% of patients. In addition, 25 patients (32.9%) were dëcompensatedë according to the oedëmato-ascitic mode. Eighteen patients (23.7%) had moderate to severe renal insufficiency, including a type 2 hëpato-rënal syndrome (SHR) in 4 cases (5.3%). Cirrhosis was also complicated by hëpato-cellular carcinoma in 10 patients (13%).

In our series, the QT interval, corrected according to the "QTc cirrhosis" formula, which would be the most appropriate formula for cirrhotic patients because of a QT-RR coefficient of independence close to 0, was prolonged in 43.5% of cases. Furthermore, we found a positive correlation between this parameter and the severity of cirrhosis as evidenced by the CHILD PUGH score (r=0.292; p=0.011) and the MELD score (r=0.329; p=0.004). These results are comparable to those reported in the literature.

Assessment of systolic function according to the WCG 2005 consensus is based on LVEF, with DS defined as LVEF<55%. Based on this definition, the prevalence of DS in our study was 5.3%, which is in agreement with the results of other studies that reported a prevalence ranging from 0 to 10%. This low prevalence could be explained by the dependence of LVEF on afterload, which is increased in cirrhotic patients. This highlights the value of studying myocardial deformation using 2D Strain, a new echocardiographic modality that is independent of load conditions. Using this technique, DS was noted in 13.1% of our patients. Our results with Strain 2D thus corroborate those of previous studies, which supported its value for early detection of alteration in systolic function even before the DS defined by LVEF calculation occurs.

On the other hand, the study of diastolic function noted the presence of a DD in 51.3% of patients according to conventional criteria. Based on the 2016 ASE recommendations, which incorporate tissue Doppler parameters in the assessment of diastolic function, a DD was found in only 32.9% of cases. Similar results have been reported in the literature. In fact, conventional parameters based on mitral flow appear to overestimate DD in cirrhotic patients, given their dependence on loading conditions. This highlights the contribution of tissue Doppler data, which are independent of these conditions.

In addition to these abnormalities, MCC is characterised by a number of morphological changes in the heart chamber, which appear to affect mainly the left cavities. In our study, 59.2% of patients had left atrial dilatation as evidenced by an index volume >34ml/m2. Furthermore, when correlating different echocardiographic parameters with cirrhosis severity scores, left atrial volume was the only echocardiographic parameter positively correlated with cirrhosis severity. These results, together with those reported in the literature, suggest that left atrial dilatation should be adopted as an important marker of MCC.

At the end of this echocardiographic evaluation, the prevalence of CMC in our series was 53.9% according to the consensus definition; it was 40.8% based on tissue Doppler and 2D Strain data. Agreement between the two definitions was moderate (kappa index equal to 0.585; p<0.001). Similar results have been reported in recently published studies, the conclusions of which suggest that these new parameters should be incorporated into the assessment of cardiac function in cirrhosis, as they are both more sensitive and more specific than conventional parameters.

In our analytical study, 3 independent predictors of MCC were identified: age (OR 1.05; CI95%: 1.003-1.103; p<0.039), female sex (OR 3.006; CI95%: 1.029-8.778; p=0.044) and CHILD PUGH score>9 (OR 4.363; CI95%: 1.328-14.331; p=0.015). Similar results were found for demographic parameters. However, the link between CMC and the severity of cirrhosis remains controversial. Indeed, some studies have confirmed that CMC, particularly DD, is significantly associated with advanced cirrhosis. However, other authors have shown that the presence of this cardiac dysfunction was independent of the severity of liver disease.

Electro-echocardiographic abnormalities are of major clinical interest in current practice. Their presence in cirrhotic patients is associated with high mortality and poor prognosis. They have been adopted by some authors as independent factors in mortality, especially after liver transplantation or the introduction of TIPS. CMC is also thought to be involved in the genesis of the hepatorenal syndrome. In our series, we noted that in univariate analysis, the presence of moderate to severe renal failure was significantly associated with CMC (p=0.004). However, we have no prospective data enabling us to establish the chronology of renal dysfunction in relation to cardiac damage. The bidirectional relationship between these two organs during cirrhosis has attracted considerable scientific interest in recent years. Recent studies have suggested that CMC contributes to the development of SHR, through altered contractility and reduced cardiac output. These data could therefore lead to a reconsideration of therapeutic strategies in the management of SHR.

At the end of this study, we propose to update the definition of CMC, by including the parameters of tissue Doppler and 2D Strain, enabling this entity to be better characterised. Given its frequency, its presence at different stages of liver disease, and its major importance in the management of cirrhosis, CMC should be systematically investigated in all cirrhotic patients. This would make it possible to anticipate the onset of SHR, avoid untimely treatments that could mask cardiac dysfunction, and selectively improve cardiac function when necessary and possible.

Admittedly, much progress has been made in understanding various aspects of MCC. However, there are still many grey areas, particularly as regards future therapeutic options. Further studies are therefore needed to identify appropriate treatments, with the potential aim of modifying the disease.

the natural history of MCC, particularly in the asymptomatic phase.

6 REFERENCES

1. Lee SS. Cardiacabnormalities in liver cirrhosis. West J Med. Nov 1989;151(5):530-5.

2. Moller S, HenriksenJH .   Cardiovascular complications of cirrhosis. Gut.   1 fisvr 2008;57(2):268-78.

3. Baik S, Fouad TR,   Lee SS. Cirrhotic cardiomyopathy. OrphanetJ   RareDis . 2007;2(1):15.

4. M0ller S, Henriksen JH. Cirrhotic cardiomyopathy. J Hepatol. 2010;53(1):179-190.

5. Meluzin J, Spinarova L, Hude P, Krejci J, Poloczkova H, Podrouzkova H, et al. Left Ventricular Mechanics in Idiopathic Dilated Cardiomyopathy: Systolic-Diastolic Coupling and Torsion. J Am Soc Echocardiogr. May 2009;22(5):486-93.

6. Otavio Mocarzel L, Bicca J, Jarske L, Oliveira T, Lanzieri P, Altenburg Gismondi R. Cirrhotic cardiomyopathy: we already know. What comes next? Dig Syst. dëc 2017; 1(1): 1-5.

7. Sampaio F. Left ventricular function assessment in cirrhosis: Current methods and future directions. World J Gastroenterol. 2016;22(1):112.

8. Rrnz-del-ArbolL. Cirrhotic cardiomyopathy. World J Gastroenterol. 2015;21(41):11502.

9. Dec GW, Kondo N, Farrell ML, Dienstag J, Cosimi AB, Semigran MJ. Cardiovascular complications following liver transplantation. Clin Transplant. dëc 1995;9(6):463-71.

10. Therapondos G, Flapan AD, Plevris JN, Hayes PC. Cardiac morbidity and mortality related to orthotopic liver transplantation. Liver Transplant Off Publ Am Assoc Study Liver Dis Int Liver Transplant Soc. dëc 2004;10(12):1441 -53.

11. Van der Linden P, Le Moine O, Ghysels M, Ortinez M, Devïere J. Pulmonary hypertension after transjugular intrahepatic portosystemic shunt: effects on right ventricular function. Hepatol Baltim Md. May 1996;23(5):982-7.

12. Azoulay D, Castaing D, Dennison A, Martino W, Eyraud D, Bismuth H. Transjugular intrahepatic portosystemic shunt worsens the hyperdynamic circulatory state of the cirrhotic patient: preliminary report of a prospective study. Hepatol Baltim Md. Jan 1994;19(1):129-32.

13. Kovacs A, Schepke M, Heller J, Schild HH, Flacke S. Short-term effects of transjugular intrahepatic shunt on cardiac function assessed by cardiac MRI: preliminary results. Cardiovasc Intervent Radiol. Apr 2010;33(2):290-6.

14. Trevisani F, Di Micoli A, Zambruni A, Biselli M, Santi V, Erroi V, et al. QT interval prolongation by acute gastrointestinal bleeding in patients with cirrhosis. Liver Int Off J Int Assoc Study Liver. nov 2012;32(10):1510-5.

15. De Pietri L, Mocchegiani F, Leuzzi C, Montalti R, Vivarelli M, Agnoletti V. Transoesophageal echocardiography during liver transplantation. World J Hepatol. 18 Oct

2015;7(23):2432-48.

16. Rrnz-del-Arbol L, Acliecar L, Serradilla R, Rodr^guez-Gand^a MA, Rivero M, Garrido E, et al. Diastolic dysfunction is a predictor of poor outcomes in patients witi cirriosis, portal iypertension, and a normal creatinine. Hepatology. nov 2013;58(5):1732-41.

17. Arroyo V, Gines P, Gerbes AL, Dudley FJ, Gentilini P, Laffi G, et al. Definition and diagnostic criteria of refractory ascites and iepatorenal syndrome in cirriosis. International Ascites Club. Hepatol Baltim Md. Jan 1996;23(1):164-76.

18. Wong F, Nadim MK, Kellum JA, Salerno F, Bellomo R, Gerbes A, et al. Working Party proposal for a revised classification system of renal dysfunction in patients with cirrhosis. Gut. 1 May 2011;60(5):702-9.

19. Levey AS, Coresi J, Balk E, Kausz AT, Levin A, Steffes MW, et al. National Kidney Foundation practice guidelines for cironic kidney disease: evaluation, classification, and stratification. Ann Intern Med. 15 Jul 2003;139(2):137-47.

20. Merkel C, Zoli M, Siringo S, van Buuren H, Magalotti D, Angeli P, et al. Prognostic indicators of risk for first variceal bleeding in cirriosis: a multicenter study in 711 patients to validate and improve tie Norti Italian Endoscopic Club (NIEC) index. Am J Gastroenterol. Oct 2000;95(10):2915-20.

21. Sarin SK, Laioti D, Saxena SP, Murtiy NS, Makwana UK. Prevalence, classification and natural iistory of gastric varices: a long-term follow-up study in 568 portal iypertension patients. Hepatol Baltim Md. Dec 1992;16(6):1343-9.

22. Lang RM, Badano LP, Mor-Avi V, Afilalo J, Armstrong A, Ernande L, et al. Recommendations for Cardiac Ciamber Quantification by Eciocardiograpiy in Adults: An Update from tie American Society of Eciocardiograpiy and tie European Association of Cardiovascular Imaging. J Am Soc Eciocardiogr. Jan 2015;28(1):1-39.e14.

23. Naguei SF, Smiseti OA, Appleton CP, Byrd BF, Dokainisi H, Edvardsen T, et al. Recommendations for tie Evaluation of Left Ventricular Diastolic Function by Eciocardiograpiy: An Update from tie American Society of Eciocardiograpiy and tie European Association of Cardiovascular Imaging. J Am Soc Eciocardiogr. Apr 2016;29(4):277-314.

24. Zambruni A, Trevisani F, Caraceni P, Bernardi M. Cardiac electropiysiological abnormalities in patients witi cirriosis. J Hepatol. May 2006;44(5):994-1002.

25. Liu H, Gaskari SA, Lee SS. Cardiac and vascular cianges in cirriosis: patiogenic mechanisms. World J Gastroenterol. 14 Feb 2006;12(6):837-42.

26. Ceolotto G, Papparella I, Sticca A, Bova S, Cavalli M, Cargnelli G, et al. An abnormal gene expression of the в-adrenergic system contributes to the pathogenesis of cardiomyopatiy in cirriotic rats. Hepatology. dec 2008;48(6):1913-23.

27. Lee SS, Marty J, Mantz J, Samain E, Braillon A, Lebrec D. Desensitization of myocardial beta-adrenergic receptors in cirrhotic rats. Hepatol Baltim Md. Sept 1990;12(3 Pt 1):481-5.

28. M0ller S, Bernardi M. Interactions of the heart and the liver. Eur Heart J. 21 Sep 2013;34(36):2804-11.

29. Gerbes AL, Remien J, Jungst D, Sauerbruch T, Paumgartner G. Evidence for downregulation of beta-2-adrenoceptors in cirrhotic patients with severe ascites. Lancet Lond Engl. 21 June 1986;1(8495):1409–11.

30. Glenn TK, Honar H, Liu H, ter Keurs HEDJ, Lee SS. Role of cardiac myofilament proteins titin and collagen in the pathogenesis of diastolic dysfunction in cirrhotic rats. J Hepatol. dëc 2011;55(6):1249–55.

31. Moezi L, Gaskari SA, Lee SS. Endocannabinoids and Liver Disease. V. Endocannabinoids as mediators of vascular and cardiac abnormalities in cirrhosis. Am J physiol-gastrointest Liver Physiol. Oct 2008;295(4):G649–53.

32. Ros J, Claria J, To-Figueras J, Planaguma A, Cejudo-Martm P, Fernandez-Varo G, et al. Endogenous cannabinoids: a new system involved in the homeostasis of arterial pressure in experimental cirrhosis in the rat. Gastroenterology. Jan 2002;122(1):85–93.

33. Yang Y-Y, Liu H, Nam SW, Kunos G, Lee SS. Mechanisms of TNFalpha-induced cardiac dysfunction in cholestatic bile duct-ligated mice: interaction between TNFalpha and endocannabinoids. J Hepatol. August 2010;53(2):298 – 306.

34. Wiest R, Groszmann RJ. The paradox of nitric oxide in cirrhosis and portal hypertension: too much, not enough. Hepatol Baltim Md. ievr 2002;35(2):478 – 91.

35. Gaskari SA, Liu H, D'Mello C, Kunos G, Lee SS. Blunted cardiac response to hemorrhage in cirrhotic rats is mediated by local macrophage-released endocannabinoids. J Hepatol. June 2015;62(6):1272–7.

36. Amirtharaj GJ, Natarajan SK, Pulimood A, Balasubramanian KA, Venkatraman A, Ramachandran A. Role of Oxygen Free Radicals, Nitric Oxide and Mitochondria in Mediating Cardiac Alterations During Liver Cirrhosis Induced by Thioacetamide. Cardiovasc Toxicol. Apr 2017;17(2):175–84.

37. Ma Z, Meddings JB, Lee SS. Membrane physical properties determine cardiac beta-adrenergic receptor function in cirrhotic rats. Am J Physiol. Jul 1994;267(1 Pt 1):G87-93.

38. Chen X, Zhang X, Kubo H, Harris DM, Mills GD, Moyer J, et al. Ca2+ influx-induced sarcoplasmic reticulum Ca2+ overload causes mitochondrial-dependent apoptosis in ventricular myocytes. Circ Res. 11 Nov 2005;97(10):1009–17.

39. Nam SW, Liu H, Wong JZ, Feng AY, Chu G, Merchant N, et al. Cardiomyocyte apoptosis contributes to pathogenesis of cirrhotic cardiomyopathy in bile duct- ligated mice. Clin Sci Lond Engl 1979. 1 Oct 2014;127(8):519–26.

40. Liu H, Ma Z, Lee SS. Contribution of nitric oxide to the pathogenesis of cirrhotic cardiomyopathy in bile duct-ligated rats. Gastroenterology. May 2000;118(5):937–44.

41. Jarkovska D, Bludovska M, Mistrova E, Krizkova V, Kotyzova D, Kubikova T, et al. Expression of classical mediators in hearts of rats with hepatic dysfunction. Can J Physiol Pharmacol. nov 2017;95(11):1351–9.

42. Chayanupatkul M, Liangpunsakul S. Cirrhotic cardiomyopathy: review of pathophysiology and treatment. Hepatol Int. Jul 2014;8(3):308–15.

43. Ward CA, Ma Z, Lee SS, Giles WR. Potassium currents in atrial and ventricular myocytes from a rat model of cirrhosis. Am J Physiol. August 1997;273(2 Pt 1):G537-544.

44. Vasavan T, Ferraro E, Ibrahim E, Dixon P, Gorelik J, Williamson C. Heart and bile acids - Clinical consequences of altered bile acid metabolism. Biochim Biophys Acta BBA - Mol Basis Dis. jan 2018;39(17)30496-9.

45. Jones DEJ, Hollingsworth K, Fattakhova G, MacGowan G, Taylor R, Blamire A, et al. Impaired cardiovascular function in primary biliary cirrhosis. Am J Physiol Gastrointest Liver Physiol. May 2010;298(5):G764-773.

46. Desai MS, Eblimit Z, Thevananther S, Kosters A, Moore DD, Penny DJ, et al. Cardiomyopathy reverses with recovery of liver injury, cholestasis and cholanemia in mouse model of biliary fibrosis. Liver Int Off J Int Assoc Study Liver. Apr 2015;35(4):1464-77.

47. M0ller S, Wiese S, Halgreen H, Hove JD. Diastolic dysfunction in cirrhosis. Heart Fail Rev. Sep 2016;21(5):599-610.

48. Liu H, Song D, Lee SS. Cirrhotic cardiomyopathy. Gastroenterol Clin Biol. Oct 2002;26(10):842-7.

49. Kelbaek H, Eriksen J, Brynjolf I, Raboel A, Lund JO, Munck O, et al. Cardiac performance in patients with asymptomatic alcoholic cirrhosis of the liver. Am J Cardiol. Oct 1984;54(7):852-6.

50. Grose RD, Nolan J, Dillon JF, Errington M, Hannan WJ, Bouchier IA, et al. Exercise-induced left ventricular dysfunction in alcoholic and non-alcoholic cirrhosis. J Hepatol. March 1995;22(3):326-32.

51. Gaskari SA, Honar H, Lee SS. Therapy insight: Cirrhotic cardiomyopathy. Nat Clin Pract Gastroenterol Hepatol. June 2006;3(6):329-37.

52. Ruiz-del-Arbol L, Monescillo A, Arocena C, Valer P, Gines P, Moreira V, et al. Circulatory function and hepatorenal syndrome in cirrhosis. Hepatol Baltim Md. August 2005;42(2):439-47.

53. Wong F. Cirrhotic cardiomyopathy. Hepatol Int. March 2009;3(1):294-304.

54. VanWagner LB, Harinstein ME, Runo JR, Darling C, Serper M, Hall S, et al. Multidisciplinary approach to cardiac and pulmonary vascular disease risk assessment in liver transplantation: An evaluation of the evidence and consensus recommendations. Am J Transplant. Jan 2018;18(1):30-42.

55. Carvalheiro F, Rodrigues C, Adrego T, Viana J, Vieira H, Seco C, et al. Diastolic Dysfunction in Liver Cirrhosis: Prognostic Predictor in Liver Transplantation? Transplant Proc. Jan 2016;48(1):128-31.

56. Sampaio F, Pimenta J, Bettencourt N, Fontes-Carvalho R, Silva AP, Valente J, et al. Systolic and diastolic dysfunction in cirrhosis: a tissue-Doppler and speckle tracking echocardiography study. Liver Int. Sep 1, 2013;33(8):1158-65.

57. Nazar A, Guevara M, Sitges M, Terra C, Sola E, Guigou C, et al. LEFT ventricular function assessed by echocardiography in cirrhosis: relationship to systemic hemodynamics and renal dysfunction. J Hepatol. 2013;58(1):51-57.

58. Merli M, Calicchia A, Ruffa A, Pellicori P, Riggio O, Giusto M, et al. Cardiac dysfunction in cirrhosis is not associated with the severity of liver disease. Eur J Intern Med. March 2013;24(2):172-6.

59. Sampaio F, Pimenta J, Bettencourt N, Fontes-Carvalho R, Silva A-P, Valente J, et al. Systolic dysfunction and diastolic dysfunction do not influence medium-term prognosis in patients with cirrhosis. Eur J Intern Med. March 2014;25(3):241-6.

60. Devi L, Malik P, Mallick J, Meher L. Study of Myocardial Dysfunction in Patients with Cirrhosis of Liver. J Adv Med Res. 10 Jan 2017;24(8):1-7.

61. Sampaio F, Pimenta J. Left ventricular function assessment in cirrhosis: Current methods and future directions. World J Gastroenterol. 7 Jan 2016;22(1):112-25.

62. Gassanov N, Caglayan E, Semmo N, Massenkeil G, Er F. Cirrhotic cardiomyopathy: A cardiologist's perspective. World J Gastroenterol WJG. 14 Nov 2014;20(42):15492-8.

63. Altekin RE, Caglar B, Karakas MS, Ozel D, Deger N, Demir I. Evaluation of subclinical left ventricular systolic dysfunction using two-dimensional speckletracking echocardiography in patients with non-alcoholic cirrhosis. Hell J Cardiol. 2014;55:402-410.

64. Kazankov K, Holland-Fischer P, Andersen NH, Torp P, Sloth E, Aagaard NK, et al. Resting myocardial dysfunction in cirrhosis quantified by tissue Doppler imaging. Liver Int Off J Int Assoc Study Liver. Apr 2011;31(4):534-40.

65. Krag A, Bendtsen F, Mortensen C, Henriksen JH, M0ller S. Effects of a single terlipressin administration on cardiac function and perfusion in cirrhosis: Eur J Gastroenterol Hepatol. sept 2010;22(9):1085-92.

66. Sampaio F, Lamata P, Bettencourt N, Alt SC, Ferreira N, Kowallick JT, et al. Assessment of cardiovascular physiology using dobutamine stress cardiovascular magnetic resonance reveals impaired contractile reserve in patients with cirrhotic cardiomyopathy. J Cardiovasc Magn Reson Off J Soc Cardiovasc Magn Reson. 2015;17:61.

67. Kim MY, Baik SK, Won CS, Park HJ, Jeon HK, Hong HI, et al. Dobutamine stress echocardiography for evaluating cirrhotic cardiomyopathy in liver cirrhosis. Korean J Hepatol. 2010;16(4):376.

68. Pozzi M, Carugo S, Boari G, Pecci V, de Ceglia S, Maggiolini S, et al. Evidence of functional and structural cardiac abnormalities in cirrhotic patients with and without ascites. Hepatol Baltim Md. Nov 1997;26(5):1131-7.

69. Finucci G, Desideri A, Sacerdoti D, Bolognesi M, Merkel C, Angeli P, et al. Left ventricular diastolic function in liver cirrhosis. Scand J Gastroenterol. March 1996;31(3):279-84.

70. Torregrosa M, Aguadë S, Dos L, Segura R, Gonzalez A, Evangelista A, et al. Cardiac alterations in cirrhosis: reversibility after liver transplantation. J Hepatol. Jan 2005;42(1):68-74.

71. Alexopoulou A, Papatheodoridis G, Pouriki S, Chrysohoou C, Raftopoulos L, Stefanadis C, et al. Diastolic myocardial dysfunction does not affect survival in patients with cirrhosis. Transpl Int Off J Eur Soc Organ Transplant. nov 2012;25(11):1174-81.

72. Papastergiou V, Skorda L, Lisgos P, Papakonstantinou N, Giakoumakis T, Ntousikos K, et al. Ultrasonographic prevalence and factors predicting left ventricular diastolic dysfunction in patients with liver cirrhosis: is there a correlation between the grade of diastolic dysfunction and the grade of liver disease? ScientificWorldJournal.

2012;2012:615057.

73. Chen Y, Chan AC, Chan S-C, Chok S-H, Sharr W, Fung J, et al. A detailed evaluation of cardiac function in cirrhotic patients and its alteration with or without liver transplantation. J Cardiol. fëvr 2016;67(2):140-6.

74. Bernardi M, Maggioli C, Dibra V, Zaccherini G. QT interval prolongation in liver cirrhosis: innocent bystander or serious threat? Expert Rev Gastroenterol Hepatol. fevr 2012;6(1):57-66.

75. Pall A, Czifra A, Vitalis Z, Papp M, Paragh G, Szabo Z. Pathophysiological and clinical approach to cirrhotic cardiomyopathy. J Gastrointestin Liver Dis. 2014;23(3):301-310.

76. Zambruni A, Di Micoli A, Lubisco A, Domenicali M, Trevisani F, Bernardi M. QT Interval Correction in Patients with Cirrhosis. J Cardiovasc Electrophysiol. Jan 2007;18(1):77-82.

77. Hansen S, M0ller S, Bendtsen F, Jensen G, Henriksen JH. Diurnal variation and dispersion in QT interval in cirrhosis: Relation to haemodynamic changes. J Hepatol. Sept 2007;47(3):373-80.

78. Li L, Liu H, Shu J, Xi X, Wang Y. [Clinical investigation of Q-T prolongation in hepatic cirrhosis]. Zhonghua Yi Xue Za Zhi. 16 Oct 2007;87(38):2717-8.

79. Genovesi S, Pizzala DMP, Pozzi M, Ratti L, Milanese M, Pieruzzi F, et al. QT interval prolongation and decreased heart rate variability in cirrhotic patients: relevance of hepatic venous pressure gradient and serum calcium. Clin Sci. 2009;116(12):851-859.

80. Bashir Bhatti A, Ali F, Akbar Satti S. Prolonged QTc Interval Is an Electrophysiological Hallmark of Cirrhotic Cardiomyopathy. Open J Intern Med. 2014;04(01):33-9.

81. Kim SM, George B, Alcivar-Franco D, Campbell CL, Charnigo R, Delisle B, et al. QT prolongation is associated with increased mortality in end-stage liver disease. World J Cardiol. 2017;9(4):347.

82. Kadappu KK, Abhayaratna K, Boyd A, French JK, Xuan W, Abhayaratna W, et al. Independent Echocardiographic Markers of Cardiovascular Involvement in Chronic Kidney Disease: The Value of Left Atrial Function and Volume. J Am Soc Echocardiogr. Apr 2016;29(4):359-67.

83. Tsang TSM, Barnes ME, Gersh BJ, Bailey KR, Seward JB. Left atrial volume as a morphophysiologic expression of left ventricular diastolic dysfunction and relation to cardiovascular risk burden. Am J Cardiol. 15 dëc 2002;90(12):1284-9.

84. Finucci G, Desideri A, Sacerdoti D, Bolognesi M, Merkel C, Angeli P, et al. Left ventricular diastolic function in liver cirrhosis. Scand J Gastroenterol. March 1996;31(3):279-84.

85. Li X, Yu S, Li L, Han D, Dai S, Gao Y. Cirrhosis-related changes in left ventricular function and correlation with the model for end-stage liver disease score. Int J Clin Exp Med. 15 dëc 2014;7(12):5751-7.

86. Merli M, Torromeo C, Giusto M, Iacovone G, Riggio O, Puddu PE. Survival at 2 years among liver cirrhotic patients is influenced by left atrial volume and left ventricular mass. Liver Int. May 2017;37(5):700-6.

87. Ortiz-Olvera NX, Castellanos-Pallares G, G6mez-Jimënez LM, Cabrera-Munoz ML,

Mëndez-Navarro J, Moran-Villota S, et al. Anatomical cardiac alterations in liver cirrhosis: an autopsy study. Ann Hepatol. 2011;10(3):321-326.

88. Lunseth JH, Olmstead EG, Abboud F. A study of heart disease in one hundred eight hospitalized patients dying with portal cirrhosis. AMA Arch Intern Med. Sept 1958;102(3):405-13.

89. Lee RF, Glenn TK, Lee SS. Cardiac dysfunction in cirrhosis. Best Pract Res Clin Gastroenterol. Jan 2007;21(1):125-40.

90. Chen Y, Chan AC, Chan S-C, Chok S-H, Sharr W, Fung J, et al. A detailed evaluation of cardiac function in cirrhotic patients and its alteration with or without liver transplantation. J Cardiol. fëvr 2016;67(2):140-6.

91. Shang C. B-type natriuretic peptide-guided therapy for perioperative medicine? Open Heart. august 2014;1(1):e000105.

92. MOller S, Bendtsen F. The pathophysiology of arterial vasodilatation and Hyperdynamic circulation in cirrhosis. Liver Int. 2018;00:1-11

93. Wong F, Siu S, Liu P, Blendis LM. Brain natriuretic peptide: is it a predictor of cardiomyopathy in cirrhosis? Clin Sci Lond Engl 1979. dëc 2001;101(6):621 -8.

94. Henriksen JH, G0tze JP, Fuglsang S, Christensen E, Bendtsen F, MOller S. Increased circulating pro-brain natriuretic peptide (proBNP) and brain natriuretic peptide (BNP) in patients with cirrhosis: relation to cardiovascular dysfunction and severity of disease. Gut. Oct 2003;52(10):1511-7.

95. Wiese S, Mortensen C, G0tze JP, Christensen E, Andersen O, Bendtsen F, et al. Cardiac and proinflammatory markers predict prognosis in cirrhosis. Liver Int. Jul 2014;34(6):e19-30.

96. Pateron D, Beyne P, Laperche T, Logeard D, Lefilliatre P, Sogni P, et al. Elevated circulating cardiac troponin I in patients with cirrhosis. Hepatol Baltim Md. March 1999;29(3):640-3.

97. Sharma UC, Pokharel S, van Brakel TJ, van Berlo JH, Cleutjens JPM, Schroen B, et al. Galectin-3 marks activated macrophages in failure-prone hypertrophied hearts and contributes to cardiac dysfunction. Circulation. 9 Nov 2004;110(19):3121-8.

98. Kimer N, Goetze JP, Bendtsen F, MOller S. New vasoactive peptides in cirrhosis: organ extraction and relation to the vasodilatory state. Eur J Clin Invest. May 2014;44(5):441-52.

99. Reant P, Labrousse L, Lafitte S, Bordachar P, Pillois X, Tariosse L, et al. Experimental Validation of Circumferential, Longitudinal, and Radial 2Dimensional Strain During Dobutamine Stress Echocardiography in Ischemic Conditions. J Am Coll Cardiol. Jan 2008;51(2):149-57.

100. Yiu KH, Schouffoer AA, Marsan NA, Ninaber MK, Stolk J, Vlieland TV, et al. Left ventricular dysfunction assessed by speckle-tracking strain analysis in patients with systemic sclerosis: Relationship to functional capacity and ventricular arrhythmias. Arthritis Rheum. dëc 2011;63(12):3969-78.

101. Zhao C-T, Yeung C-K, Siu C-W, Tam S, Chan J, Chen Y, et al. Relationship between parathyroid hormone and subclinical myocardial dysfunction in patients with severe psoriasis. J Eur Acad Dermatol Venereol. Apr 2014;28(4):461-8.

102. Chen Y, Chung H-Y, Zhao C-T, Wong A, Zhen Z, Tsang HH-L, et al. Left

ventricular myocardial dysfunction and premature atherosclerosis in patients with axial spondyloarthritis. Rheumatology. fisvr 2015;54(2):292-301.

103.	Lang RM, Badano LP, Mor-Avi V, Afilalo J, Armstrong A, Ernande L, et al. Recommendations for cardiac chamber quantification by echocardiography in adults: an update from the American Society of Echocardiography and the European Association of Cardiovascular Imaging. J Am Soc Echocardiogr Off Publ Am Soc Echocardiogr. Jan 2015;28(1):1-39.e14.

104.	Nazar A, Guevara M, Sitges M, Terra C, Sola E, Guigou C, et al. LEFT ventricular function assessed by echocardiography in cirrhosis: relationship to systemic hemodynamics and renal dysfunction. J Hepatol. 2013;58(1):51-57.

105.	Sampaio F, Pimenta J, Bettencourt N, Fontes-Carvalho R, Silva AP, Valente J, et al. Systolic and diastolic dysfunction in cirrhosis: a tissue-Doppler and speckle tracking echocardiography study. Liver Int. Sep 2013;33(8):1158-65.

106.	Nagueh SF, Appleton CP, Gillebert TC, Marino PN, Oh JK, Smiseth OA, et al. Recommendations for the Evaluation of Left Ventricular Diastolic Function by Echocardiography. Eur J Echocardiogr. August 4, 2008;10(2):165-93.

107.	Nagueh SF, Smiseth OA, Appleton CP, Byrd BF, Dokainish H, Edvardsen T, et al. Recommendations for the Evaluation of Left Ventricular Diastolic Function by Echocardiography: An Update from the American Society of Echocardiography and the European Association of Cardiovascular Imaging. J Am Soc Echocardiogr. Apr 2016;29(4):277-314.

108.	Cahill JM, Horan M, Quigley P, Maurer B, McDonald K. Doppler-echocardiographic indices of diastolic function in heart failure admissions with preserved left ventricular systolic function. Eur J Heart Fail. August 2002;4(4):473-8.

109.	Palmieri V, Innocenti F, Pini R, Celentano A. Reproducibility of Doppler echocardiographic assessment of left ventricular diastolic function in multicenter setting. J Am Soc Echocardiogr Off Publ Am Soc Echocardiogr. fèvr 2005;18(2):99-106.

110.	Petrie MC, Hogg K, Caruana L, McMurray JJV. Poor concordance of commonly used echocardiographic measures of left ventricular diastolic function in patients with suspected heart failure but preserved systolic function: is there a reliable echocardiographic measure of diastolic dysfunction? Heart Br Card Soc. May 2004;90(5):511-7.

111.	Thomas MD, Fox KF, Wood DA, Gibbs JSR, Coats AJS, Henein MY, et al. Echocardiographic features and brain natriuretic peptides in patients presenting with heart failure and preserved systolic function. Heart Br Card Soc. May 2006;92(5):603-8.

112.	Klein AL, Burstow DJ, Tajik AJ, Zachariah PK, Bailey KR, Seward JB. Effects of age on left ventricular dimensions and filling dynamics in 117 normal persons. Mayo Clin Proc. March 1994;69(3):212-24.

113.	Nagueh SF, Appleton CP, Gillebert TC, Marino PN, Oh JK, Smiseth OA, et al. Recommendations for the evaluation of left ventricular diastolic function by echocardiography. Eur J Echocardiogr J Work Group Echocardiogr Eur Soc Cardiol. March 2009;10(2):165-93.

114.	Somani PO, contractor Q, Chaurasia AS, Rathi PM. Diastolic dysfunction characterizes cirrhotic cardiomyopathy. Indian Heart J. 2014;66(6):649-55.

115. Karagiannakis DS, Vlachogiannakos J, Anastasiadis G, Vafiadis-Zouboulis I, Ladas SD. Diastolic cardiac dysfunction is a predictor of dismal prognosis in patients with liver cirrhosis. Hepatol Int. Oct 2014;8(4):588-94.

116. Falletta C, Fili D, Nugara C, Di Gesaro G, Mina C, Baravoglia CMH, et al. Diastolic dysfunction diagnosed by tissue Doppler imaging in cirrhotic patients: Prevalence and its possible relationship with clinical outcome. Eur J Intern Med. dëc 2015;26(10):830-4.

117. Rimba§ RC, Baldea SM, Guerra RDGA, Visoiu SI, Rimba§ M, Pop CS, et al. New Definition Criteria of Myocardial Dysfunction in Patients with Liver Cirrhosis: A Speckle Tracking and Tissue Doppler Imaging Study. Ultrasound Med Biol. Jan 2018;44(3):562-574.

118. Pozzi M, Redaelli E, Ratti L, Poli G, Guidi C, Milanese M, et al. Time-course of diastolic dysfunction in different stages of chronic HCV related liver diseases. Minerva Gastroenterol Dietol. June 2005;51(2):179-86.

119. Salerno F, Gerbes A, Gines P, Wong F, Arroyo V. Diagnosis, prevention and treatment of hepatorenal syndrome in cirrhosis. Gut. Sept 2007;56(9):1310-8.

120. de Mattos AZ, de Mattos AA, Mëndez-Sanchez N. Hepatorenal syndrome: Current concepts related to diagnosis and management. Ann Hepatol. august 2016;15(4):474-81.

121. Ruiz-del-Arbol L, Serradilla R. Cirrhotic cardiomyopathy. World J Gastroenterol. 7 Nov 2015;21(41):11502-21.

122. Ruiz-del-Arbol L, Urman J, Fernandez J, Gonzalez M, Navasa M, Monescillo A, et al. Systemic, renal, and hepatic hemodynamic derangement in cirrhotic patients with spontaneous bacterial peritonitis. Hepatol Baltim Md. Nov 2003;38(5):1210-8.

123. Krag A, Bendtsen F, Henriksen JH, M0ller S. Low cardiac output predicts development of hepatorenal syndrome and survival in patients with cirrhosis and ascites. Gut. Jan 2010;59(1):105-10.

124. Mocarzel LO, Bicca J, Jarske L, Oliveira T, Lanzieri P, Gismondi R, et al. Cirrhotic Cardiomyopathy: Another Case of a Successful Approach to Treatment of Hepatorenal Syndrome. Case Rep Gastroenterol. dëc 2016;10(3):531 -7.

125. Zardi EM, Abbate A, Zardi DM, Dobrina A, Margiotta D, Van Tassel BW, et al. Cirrhotic Cardiomyopathy. J Am Coll Cardiol. August 2010;56(7):539-49.

126. Albarmawi A, Czock D, Gauss A, Ehehalt R, Lorenzo Bermejo J, Burhenne J, et al. CYP3A activity in severe liver cirrhosis correlates with Child-Pugh and model for end-stage liver disease (MELD) scores: CYP3A activity and severity of liver cirrhosis. Br J Clin Pharmacol. Jan 2014;77(1):160-9.

127. Vuphalanchi R, Liang T, Goswami CP, Nalamasu R, Li L, Jones D, et al. Relationship between Differential Hepatic microRNA Expression and Decreased Hepatic Cytochrome P450 3A Activity in Cirrhosis. Ray R, ë editor. PLoS ONE. 13 Sep 2013;8(9):e74471.

128. Di Micoli A, Zambruni A, Bracci E, Benazzi B, Zappoli P, Berzigotti A, et al. "Torsade de pointes" during amiodarone infusion in a cirrhotic woman with a prolonged QT interval. Dig Liver Dis. Jul 2009;41(7):535-8.

129. Werner C, Riessen R, Gregor M, Bitzer M. Unerwartete Komplikation nach Osophagusvarizenblutung - Fall 2/2011. DMW - Dtsch Med Wochenschr. ievr

2011;136(05):217-217.

130.   Lehmann M, Bruns T, Herrmann A, Fritzenwanger M, Stallmach A. 54-jahriger Patient mit Leberzirrhose und therapiebedingten Torsade-de-pointes-Tachykardien. Internist. Apr 2011;52(4):445-50.

131.   Letsas KP, Efremidis M, Filippatos GS, Sideris AM. Drug-induced long QT syndrome. Hell J Cardiol HJC Hell Kardiologike Epitheorese. Oct 2007;48(5):296-9.

132.   Santeusanio AD, Dunsky KG, Pan S, Schiano TD. The Impact of Cirrhosis and Prescription Medications on QTc Interval Before and After Liver Transplantation. J Pharm Pract. nov 2017;089719001773789.

133.   Cazzaniga M, Salerno F, Pagnozzi G, Dionigi E, Visentin S, Cirello I, et al. Diastolic dysfunction is associated with poor survival in patients with cirrhosis with transjugular intrahepatic portosystemic shunt. Gut. 1 June 2007;56(6):869-75.

134.   Mittal C, Qureshi W, Singla S, Ahmad U, Huang MA. Pre-transplant left ventricular diastolic dysfunction is associated with post transplant acute graft rejection and graft failure. Dig Dis Sci. March 2014;59(3):674-80.

135.   Dowsley TF, Bayne DB, Langnas AN, Dumitru I, Windle JR, Porter TR, et al. Diastolic dysfunction in patients with end-stage liver disease is associated with development of heart failure early after liver transplantation. Transplantation. 27 Sep 2012;94(6):646-51.

136.   Tandon M, Karna ST, Pandey CK, Chaturvedi R. Diagnostic and therapeutic challenge of heart failure after liver transplant: Case series. World J Hepatol. 28 Nov 2017;9(33):1253-60.

137.   Eimer MJ, Wright JM, Wang EC, Kulik L, Blei A, Flamm S, et al. Frequency and significance of acute heart failure following liver transplantation. Am J Cardiol. 2008 Jan 15;101(2):242-4.

138.   Mandell MS, Seres T, Lindenfeld J, Biggins SW, Chascsa D, Ahlgren B, et al. Risk factors associated with acute heart failure during liver transplant surgery: a case control study. Transplantation. Apr 2015;99(4):873-8.

139.   Somani PO, contractor Q, Chaurasia AS, Rathi PM. Diastolic dysfunction characterizes cirrhotic cardiomyopathy. Indian Heart J. Nov 2014;66(6):649-55.

140.   Bernardi M, Maggioli C, Dibra V, Zaccherini G. QT interval prolongation in liver cirrhosis: innocent bystander or serious threat? Expert Rev Gastroenterol Hepatol. 1 Feb 2012;6(1):57-66.

141.   Cesari M, Frigo AC, Tonon M, Angeli P. ardiovascular predictors of death in patients with cirrhosis. Hepatology.Sep 13, 2017; 6(47):1527-3350.

142.   Dadhich S, Goswami A, Jain VK, Gahlot A, Kulamarva G, Bhargava N. Cardiac dysfunction in cirrhotic portal hypertension with or without ascites. Ann Gastroenterol Q Publ Hell Soc Gastroenterol. 2014;27(3):244.

143.   Henriksen JH, Bendtsen F, Hansen EF, M0ller S. Acute non-selective β-adrenergic blockade reduces prolonged frequency-adjusted Q-T interval (QTc) in patients with cirrhosis. J Hepatol. Feb 2004;40(2):239-46.

144.   Zardi EM, Abbate A, Zardi DM, Dobrina A, Margiotta D, Van Tassel BW, et al. Cirrhotic cardiomyopathy. J Am Coll Cardiol. August 2010;56(7):539-49.

145.   Cheng CP, Igarashi Y, Little WC. Mechanism of increased rate of left ventricular

filling during exercise. Circ Res. Jan 1992;70(1):9-19.

146.   Serste T, Francoz C, Durand F, Rautou P-E, Melot C, Valla D, et al. Beta-blockers cause paracentesis-induced circulatory dysfunction in patients with cirrhosis and refractory ascites: a cross-over study. J Hepatol. Oct 2011;55(4):794-9.

147.   Baik S, Fouad TR, Lee SS. Cirrhotic cardiomyopathy. Orphanet J Rare Dis. 2007;2(1):15.

148.   Pozzi M, Carugo S, Boari G, Pecci V, de Ceglia S, Maggiolini S, et al. Evidence of functional and structural cardiac abnormalities in cirrhotic patients with and without ascites. Hepatol Baltim Md. Nov 1997;26(5):1131-7.

149.   Torregrosa M, Aguade S, Dos L, Segura R, Gonzalez A, Evangelista A, et al. Cardiac alterations in cirrhosis: reversibility after liver transplantation. J Hepatol. Jan 2005;42(1):68-74.

150.   Sonny A, Govindarajan SR, Jaber WA, Cywinski JB. Systolic heart failure after liver transplantation: Incidence, predictors, and outcome. Clin Transplant. 1 Feb 2018;e13199.

APPENDIX 1: OUTLINE OF THE THESIS

Last name   :;   **First name**   :;   **D NUMBER** : ;

Age :

Sex : Male ___[]_;   Female [_____]

ATCD : diabete O ; dyslipidëmie 1   ; Other :

Medication taken: beta blockers   , _____ diuretics   ;

Other :_____||___[_____]

Habits: Alcohol   ; Tobacco   (PA=)

Discovery tours :   O

icterus abdominal pain

Ascites _____11   hëdigestive bleeding 11   ëabdominal ultrasound O

Disturbance of the l^patic balanceQ   thrombopënie[ )

Others :

Characteristics of cirrhosis :

Etiology: HBV[1HCV _||_CBP [1CSP |_   1Sd overlap __|1

NASH □ CBS O   Budd Chiari O cryptogënique O

Sëvëritë : CHILD   PUGH=MELD=

Evolving complications: Hëdigestive bleeding [___]   number of episodes :

DOA □ number of episode(s) :

CHC □ EHQ   SHR □

FOGD data: VO absentOC IIO IIIO

VG   absentQGOV1 ⊓   GOVCIGV1QIGV2 O

GHTP □ **Abdominal ultrasound data:** SMG |1fleche sptenique=

CVC □Dilatation   TPQ

Biological data : Hb :; plaq=; ASAT=   ;   ALAT= .

BD/BT=   /GGT= ; PAL= ;   Albumin=

TP= ; INR=   ; uree=;   creat= ;   Na+/K+=.../....

Clinical data :

Weight=   ; Height=

TA= ; Fc=

Ascites □OMI □

ECG :   QT]= [QT

Other anomaly(ies) :

APPENDIX 2: CHILD-PUGH SCORE

Points	1	2	3
Ascites	absent	moderee	abundant
Hepatic encephalopathy	absent	Stages 1 and 2	Stages 3 and 4
Prothrombin rate(%)	>50	50-40	<40
Total bilirubin(umol/l)	<35	35-50	>50
Albumin(g/l)	>35	28-35	<28

Stage A : Score=5-6points
Stage B : Score=7-9points
Stace C: Score > 10-15 points

APPENDIX 3: MELD SCORE

MELD score = 3.8 **x** In **[**Bilirubinemia (in mg/dL)**]** + 11.2 **x** In (INR) + 9.6 **x** In**[**Creatinemia (in mg/dL)**]** + 6.4

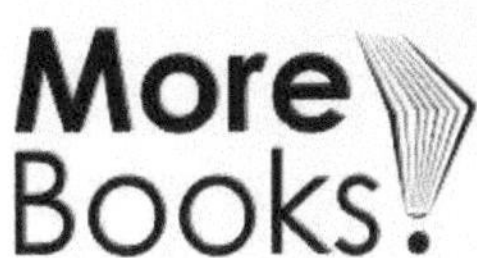

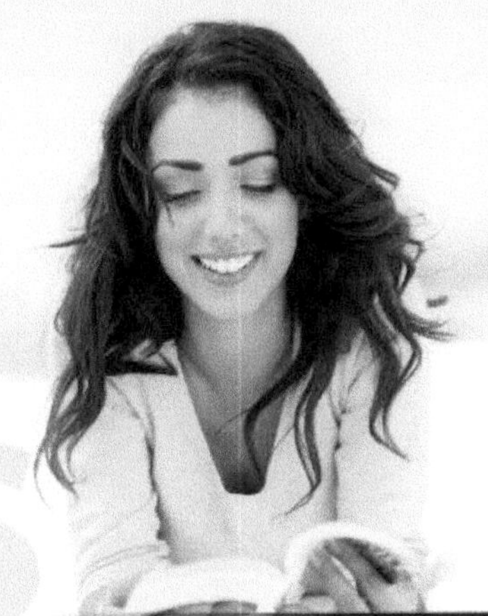

I want morebooks!

Buy your books fast and straightforward online - at one of world's fastest growing online book stores! Environmentally sound due to Print-on-Demand technologies.

Buy your books online at
www.morebooks.shop

Kaufen Sie Ihre Bücher schnell und unkompliziert online – auf einer der am schnellsten wachsenden Buchhandelsplattformen weltweit! Dank Print-On-Demand umwelt- und ressourcenschonend produziert.

Bücher schneller online kaufen
www.morebooks.shop

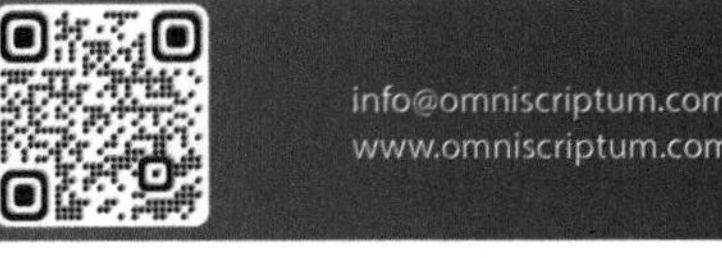

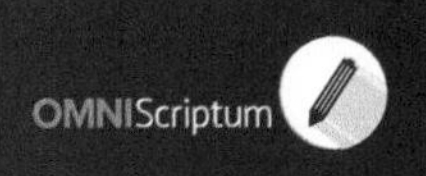

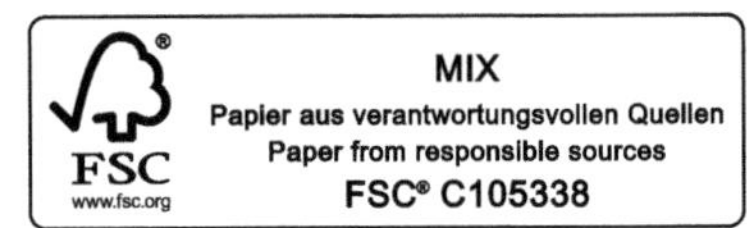

Printed by Books on Demand GmbH, Norderstedt / Germany